D1532694

Calorie Accounting

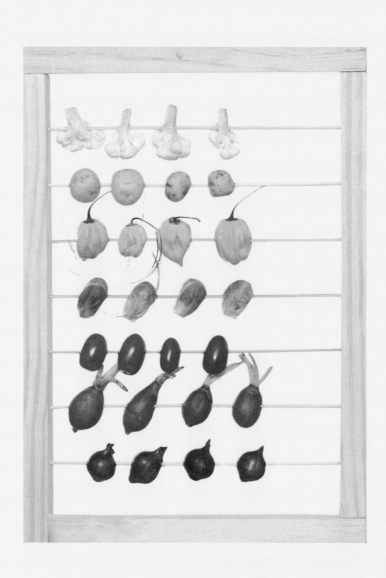

Calorie Accounting

THE FOOLPROOF DIET-BY-NUMBERS PLAN FOR A SKINNIER NEW YOU

MANDY LEVY

Skyhorse Publishing

Skyhorse Publishing books may be purchased in bulk at special discounts for sales promotion, corporate gifts, fund-raising, or educational purposes. Special editions can also be created to specifications. For details, contact the Special Sales Department, Skyhorse Publishing, 307 West 36th Street, 11th Floor, New York, NY 10018 or info@skyhorsepublishing.com.

Skyhorse® and Skyhorse Publishing® are registered trademarks of Skyhorse Publishing, Inc.®, a Delaware corporation.

Visit our website at www.skyhorsepublishing.com.

10 9 8 7 6 5 4 3 2 1

Library of Congress Cataloging-in-Publication Data is available on file.

Cover design by Rain Saukas
Cover photo credit: Christopher Patrick Ernst

Print ISBN: 978-1-63220-472-1
Ebook ISBN: 978-1-63220-797-5

Printed in China

For Mom and Dad. Y'all cray. LY.

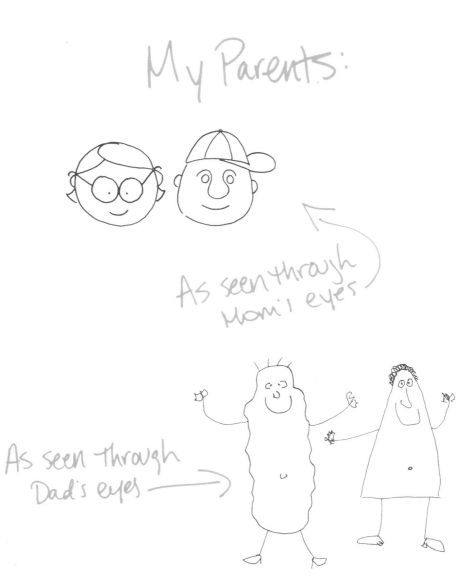

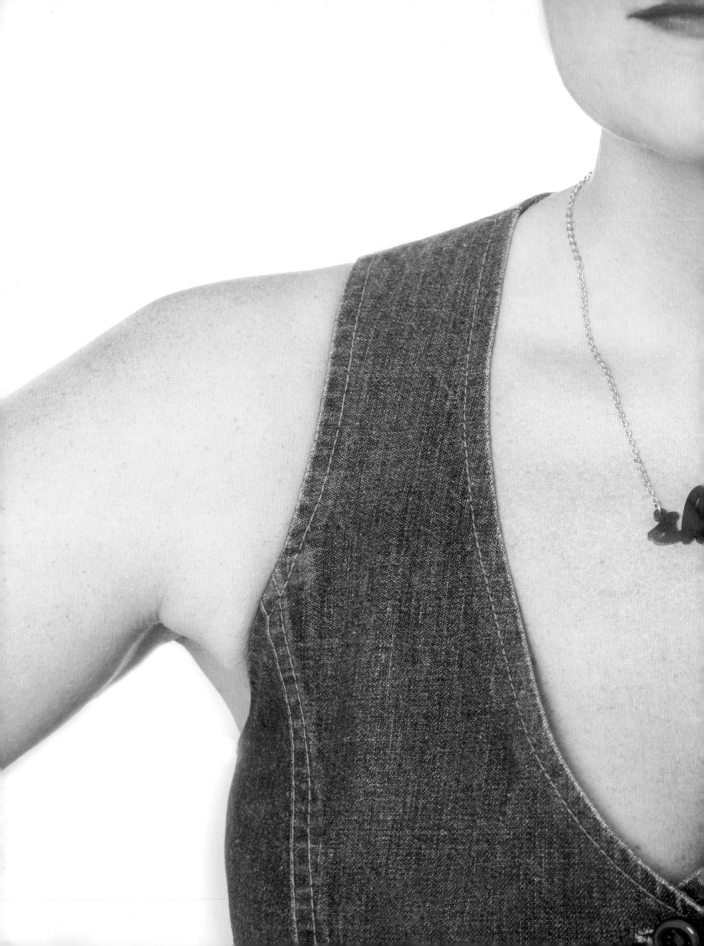

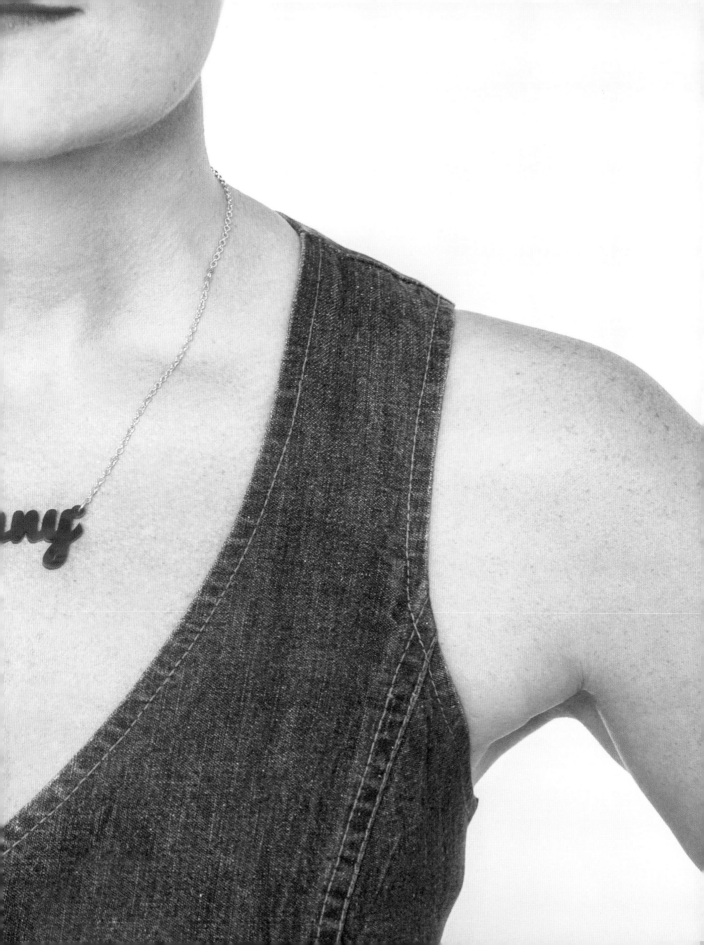

CONTENTS

Disclaimer

Any fatty who is considering buying this book needs to make sure they can put that thick skin to some good use. We're trying to get skinny here, people, and we don't have time to get butt-hurt about feelings or sensitive about political correctness, bullying, egos, errant jabs at vegans and/or yoga, etc. Dieting sucks—we all know that. But attitude is everything, and success can be a long-ish journey. The least you can do is have a little fun getting there. If the Doughboy can giggle when someone pokes at his rolls, so can you. The fact of the matter is this: You're heavy. So do yourself a favor and lighten up!

Also, I am not a doctor. I'm just some schmuck like you.

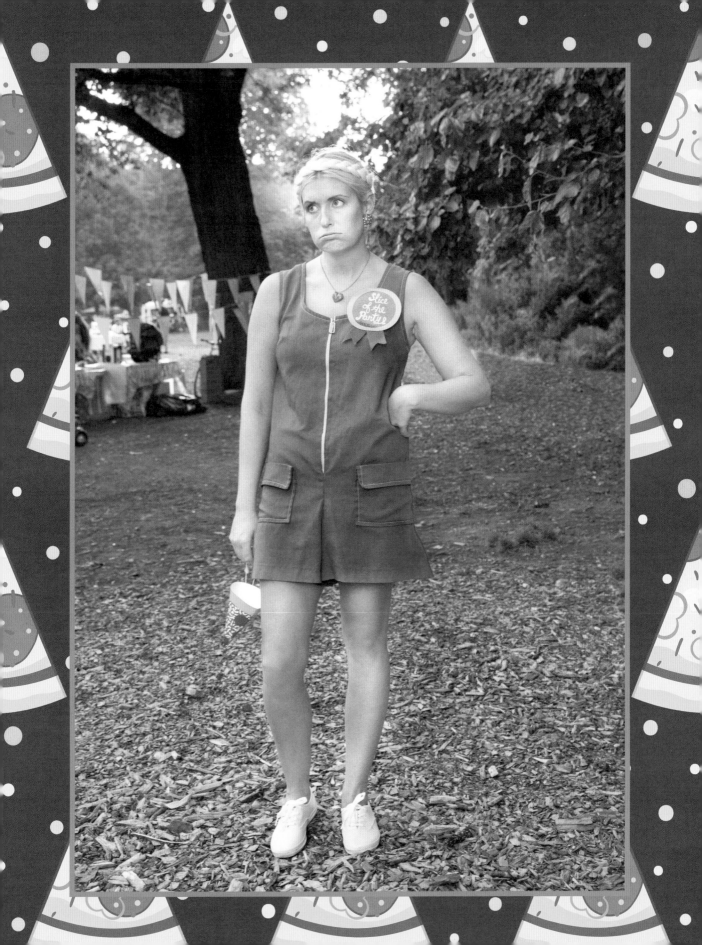

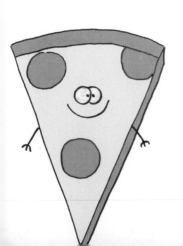

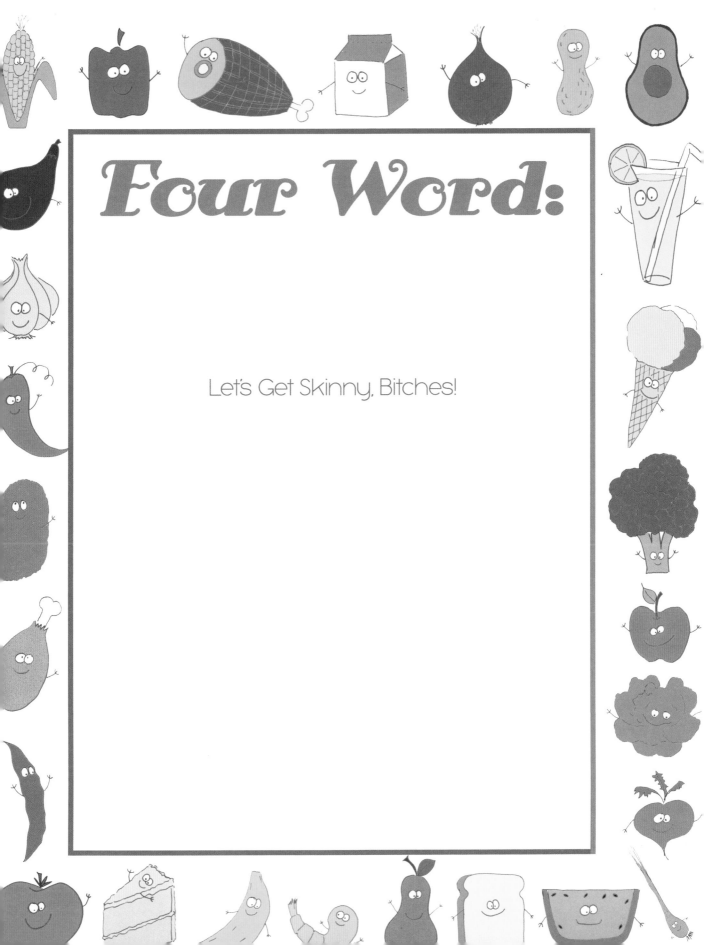

Four Word:

Let's Get Skinny, Bitches!

Foreword

Well howdy-ho, plump dumpling! Fancy meeting you here, in the perpetually euphemized Health & Fitness section of your local bookseller's shoppe! I can tell just looking at you that you're neither healthy nor fit, but baby beluga, that's what I'm here for. Super snaps for conquering the first step: admitting you have a problem, and deciding to do something about it. That part sucks, so good for you! And from what I can see, you're a perfectly human sort of being with hands and eyes and impeccable taste, and perhaps you've just let that impeccable taste get the better of you over the months, or years, or decades, or whatever. The point is, you're fat. Maybe it's the freshman fifteen, maybe you just gave birth to triplets, maybe you make yourself a pan of brownies every morning for breakfast. Whatever the reason, you're fat. And you'd rather you weren't. You've tried all the fad diets, flirted with all the fashionable disorders, spent hundreds on miracle pills, but in the end, Miracle Whip has been your only friend. The beautiful clothes that hang in your closet, price tags still attached, are collecting dust. Your Facebook profile pic is over two years old. You haven't felt the gentle touch of a lover since . . . never mind. But now you're determined, once and for all, to squeeze that fine ass into those skinny jeans and strut the streets like they're your runway. You just need to know that *this* time will be *the* time. You just need to know it will work. Well, I may not have Dr. Atkins and Suzanne Somers and *The Today Show* dieticians proving my sciences, but I'm pretty sure Einstein would have my back. Calorie Accounting, boys and girls, is math. It's simple arithmetic. Black and white. Right and wrong. No guessing, just knowing. Just fact. This time, it will work. Everybody bring a calculator?

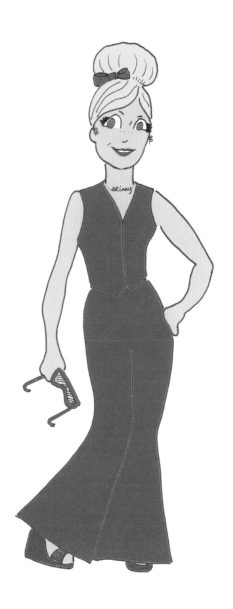

Introduction:
Well Who the Hell Are You?

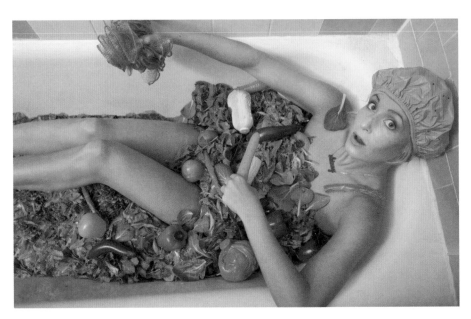

Valid question.

Perhaps this clever poem I often employed to vandalize the chalkboards of various junior high classrooms will help clear things up:

Mandy is awesome,
Mandy is the best,
Mandy is better than all the rest!

Do you trust me yet? Well, I suppose I can cough up a little more detail.

My name is Mandy Levy. I'm 31, and I've been lying about my age for 3 years now. That was the first time in a long time I've told the truth. (Or was it?) It was. I like to consider my life thus far a "try-coastal" experiment.

Born to the Chicago shores of Lake Michigan, I made the most of my Midwestern upbringing and education. I have distinct memories of waking up in the mornings before high school, thinking to myself, *I sure am lucky to be so perfect.* I was student council president, head of the class, *not* on the goddamn homecoming court (but who's really dwelling on that?), and a champion golfer and badminton player. And no, that's nowhere near as horrifying as it appears typed out on paper. I was blonde enough and thin enough (teenage metabolism is not something to take for granted, people!) to be admired and oftentimes stalked by staggering numbers of hearing-impaired and/or sweaty-handed exchange students at school, which only encouraged me. Even after four years of angst and rebellion and forced intellectualism in college I was still so taken with my highly developed superiority complex that immediately upon graduation I flew my delusions out to Hollywood to "make it." The most I made was a $60 tip at Maggiano's, and on Tuesdays I sat in Judge Judy's jury as a professional audience member, rubbing shoulders with the other junkies and vagrants who agreed to a ten-hour day on set with the promise of Oreos, cigarette breaks, and $6.75 an hour. Oh, I was a star.

And like any struggling young starlet might, in order to dull the pain of failure, I turned to the drink. And the food. And the more food. And because my résumé didn't tout much more than a voiceover for a chronic constipation commercial, I wasn't really a frontrunner for *Dr. Drew's Celebrity Rehab*. I got fat. And so I went back home to the Midwest, where at least I'd blend in.

I spent four years in Cincinnati, Ohio. Respectfully, some of the most fun and most productive years of my life. I met wonderful people, fell in love with the city, won an Emmy (google me, I'm serious!), founded a successful arts and events collective, and became something of a small-town society girl, if I do say so myself (and I do). But widespread adoration and tangible success did not feed me enough. My confidence was up but so was my dress size. I paid the price for all the partying, stumbling home every night at 3:00 a.m., having become the unofficial spokesperson for the Taco Bell "Fourthmeal" campaign, and soon I was a cow-and-a-half, even by Midwestern standards, and cows are, like, an industry there.

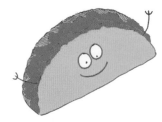

I tried anorexia but liked food too much. Tried bulimia but I was way too lazy and only ever got as far as the bingeing part. Tried Atkins but I missed pasta, tried Weight Watchers but lost my patience, tried a three-week liquid cleanse and was impressed with an initial thirteen-pound loss but quite depressed after one bite of celebratory solid food instantly packed twenty pounds of cellulite onto my ass. I tried a personal trainer but wanted to strangle her, tried the Zone but went cross-eyed, tried Nutrisystem but went broke, and was just about to try crystal meth but I realized my face might turn out like Fergie's so I threw up my hands. I got myself another beer and ate a block of cheese.

I had lost myself. I wasn't happy. I was partied out and needed to grow up. I needed to be *me* again—get that glowing superiority complex back. I needed to look at my life and recognize what I had—a love of money, a love of shopping, and love handles—and apply it to what I wanted—more money, more clothes, and a hot bod that could rightly flaunt these attributes. So I took the only logical next step: dropped everything, moved to New York City, cooped myself up for six months of solitude in a Brooklyn cocoon, set my mind to the metamorphosis at hand, and now poof! I'm a motherfucking butterfly. I've lost thirty-five pounds and counting. I look good, I feel good . . . I'm a self-made Mandy. I gotta tell you guys, I've invented a freaking genius diet plan here. It's such a relief: it's so easy, so rewarding . . . it's even kinda fun! Feels like I've struck gold. And I want to share my riches with the world.

Calorie Accounting is the weight loss plan I've developed, and it incorporates the best practices of all the diets I've tried (and generally failed at), but then peppers in a little logic, and, as you will find, a lot of liberation. For a rather right-brained creative person, this is the most left-brained approach to anything I think I've ever taken, and, boy, has it been a comfort. Numbers are what they are. Arithmetic is what it is. You do the math and you can't get it wrong! It just absolutely, positively 100 percent will work. No more hypotheses about the effectiveness of an electroshock belly belt or an acai berry. No more impatient, unsatisfied trial runs in the front-row car of the fad diet rollercoaster. No more misery of tagging along with a plan that doesn't feel right because it simply wasn't built for you. With Calorie Accounting, you're running your own business. You're managing your own balance. *You* are the boss, *you* roll out the budget, *you* control the spending, and eventually, *you* reap all the benefits of a fortune that will surely come with a little patience, self-control, and education in the marketplace. So are you ready to start financing your figure? Then read on, my little chubby wubby. Read on.

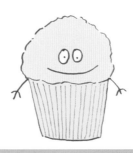

Calorieconomics 101

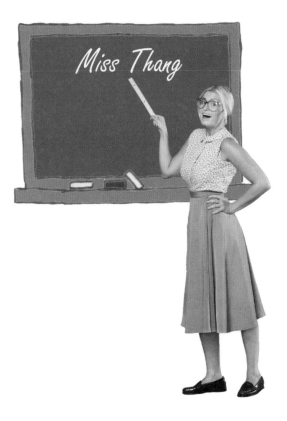

Miss Thang

Good morning, class, and welcome to Calorieconomics 101. I'm your teacher, Miss Thang, and—
Sweet jezebel, Billy, get that eraser out of your ear! Miranda, get that pencil out of your nose! And Carl, get that finger out of your—
Hmph. As I was saying. This is Calorieconomics. Prepare to get schooled.

The Equation of Equations of Equations

How do I not be fat? Since the beginning of time, the age-old answer to that age-old question is older than ages: *Eat less, exercise more.* Yes, but what does that mean, exactly? *Be less of a hog, be more of a sweat.* That didn't help. *Take in less than you put out.* Are you calling me a slut? Okay, let's start over.

A calorie is defined as one unit of energy. This is the energy we require to fuel our bodies and stay alive. We also need this energy to expend on "work," which is any life activity outside the confines of being a bedridden vegetable. Like gasoline to a semi, we humans must guzzle and emit calories regularly in order to "keep on truckin'."

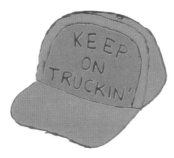

Now, here's where things get interesting. While one calorie equals one unit of energy, 3,500 calories equals one pound. This bears repeating.

3,500 calories = 1 pound

This means, then, if losing weight is all about calories in versus calories out, all we have to do in order to lose one pound is simply create a **deficit** of 3,500 calories in a given period of time.

Did I lose anyone?

So. Say I want to drop one pound in a week. A safe and attainable goal, and we'll take it one day at a time. (Some of you know what *that* means—eh? eh?) There are three numbers I'm going to need to work with:

1. **Calories In**
2. **Calories Out**
3. **BMR**

Let's start with the first one. **Calories In.** This is the sum of all things you scarf, slurp, or snort down in a day. Everything you can ingest, even laundry detergent, I'm sure, has a caloric value assigned to it. We'll talk more about these numbers and how to track them later on, but for now, let's just say I ate 1,400 calories on this particular day. Pretty typical.

Next. **Calories Out.** It can be difficult to calculate an exact value for this one, but I've got all sorts of insider tools and tips to get you right in the ballpark. But in this example, say I was too lazy to go to the gym but I walked to and from work, a half mile each way. We'll call it an exertion of 100 calories.

And last. The savior! The **BMR.** This stands for "basal metabolic rate," and you will learn to love this number. This value indicates the amount of calories your body burns in a day, just existing. Just lying in bed, breathing, watching *Wild Hogs*. This number is also equivalent to the calories you can net in a day and maintain your weight. (That sounded like level 201 jargon. We'll get to it.) The BMR is different for everyone, and it's variable—it fluctuates as your weight, age, and/or gender might change. We'll all calculate our basal metabolic rates together in a bit and it will be super fun, but to keep focused on our example above, let's just say I'm running a BMR of 1,500 right now.

So. Let's take a closer look at our day:

1. Calories In = 1,400
2. Calories Out = 100
3. BMR = 1,500

And now here is The Equation of Equations of Equations, if you smarty-pantses haven't already figured it out:

Calories In – Calories Out – BMR = Total Net Calories

So what did we net? Well, 1,400-100-1,500 = -200. We have created a *deficit* of 200 calories today. Good, but not great. If we want to achieve a total deficit of 3,500 calories (1 pound) in one week, or 7 days, that means we'll have to average a deficit of 500 calories each day. We've fallen 300 short.

So, what change can we make tomorrow? As you cannot manually affect your BMR, you've got Calories In and Calories Out to work with. Between the two of them, you have to find a way to subtract another 300 calories from your daily total. This could mean a three-mile power walk on the treadmill in the morning, a little more willpower at dessert time, or a healthy combination of the two. We'll dive more into the solution later. But now, you finally have the equation for The Problem. You're welcome.

Now it's time to find your BMR. Where is it? Under your pillow? Behind your ear? In your belly button? No, silly, it's on the internet! (Seriously. Want to make this easy on yourself? Go to calorieaccounting.com, click on the BMR calculator, plug in some numbers, and be on your way.) But for those traditionalists and/or Canadian ex-pats who are just itching to perform metric conversions every chance they get, be my guest and go for the longhand! (Got mass decimals? Do yourself a solid and round up.)*

BMR Calculation for Women:
447.593 + (9.247 x weight in kg) + (3.098 x height in cm) - (4.330 x age in years)

BMR Calculation for Men:
88.362 + (13.397 x weight in kg) + (4.799 x height in cm) - (5.677 x age in years)

Got it? Got your Basal Metabolic Rate? AWESOME!!!!!!!!!!! That's you! That's your number! Now remember what this means: this number denotes the amount of calories your body burns in a day, sitting on the couch with your finger up your nose. Think of it as your **net worth**. Congrats! This is the first nugget of your fortune, and now you are ready to make your investment and get rich! Or thin! Or both!

---

* Never heard of the metric system? Don't rule it out! Feel free to convert to American sensibility like so: multiply inches by 2.54 to get centimeters and divide pounds by 2.2 to get kilograms. Don't forget! Your BMR changes as your weight does, so make sure to recalculate as you lose!

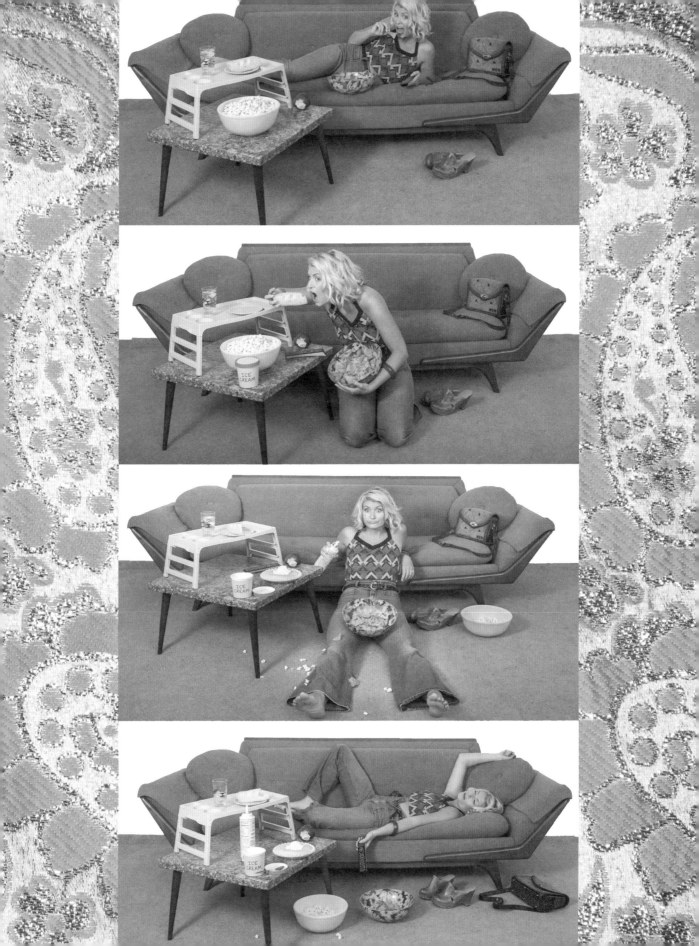

A Calorie Saved is a Calorie Earned

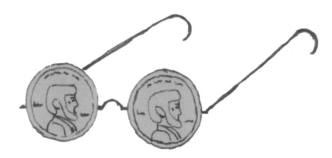

I believe it was our be-loved and be-lectrocuted founding father Benjamin Franklin who once said, "A penny saved is a penny earned". . . and that dude made bank! And what's a penny but a unit of measurement? Same goes for a calorie. Let's take his lesson in finance and apply it to our efforts in fitness.

Calories as Currency

Buy. Sell. Trade.

Since the beginning of time, these are the fundamentals that have helped shape society and human connectivity as we know it. We have some things. We want other things. It's a matter of slapping a value on those two truths to achieve some degree of satisfaction for all parties involved. From Pocahontas swapping pelts with raccoons, to the Tooth Fairy leaving a buck for a pocketful of molars, to the invention of the greatest technology known to man, eBay, this has always been and will always be our operating system. Greenbacks, cheese, big ones, smackers, lira, yen, and Australian dollars. These are the things we call money. This is currency. And now, it's time to put your money where your mouth is. For real.

In thinking of calories as currency, a few things should be noted:

1. The calories suddenly have real utilitarian value. They're good for something. They mean something. They are assets. They can be spent and saved and stretched to their limits.
2. The idea of the *new calorie*, then, should encourage a kind of greed within you. And greed, as my biological father Michael Douglas (I'm 90% sure of this) will tell you, is good.

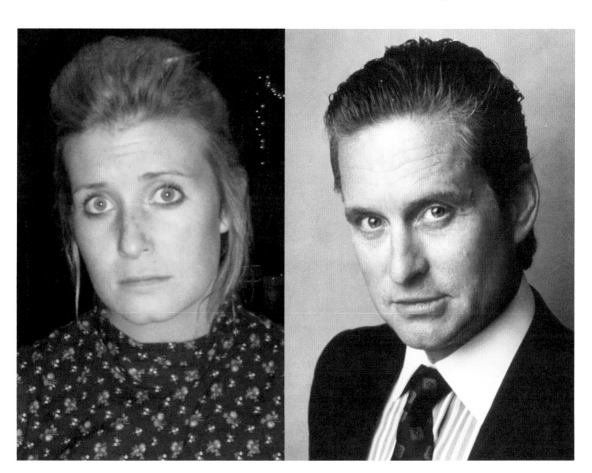

3. You will have a greater respect for the calories that come in and out of your day-to-day. They are, in both their negative and positive values, the product of your efforts. Your hard-earned pay. You will handle them with caution and care. You will be mindful of the ways you manage them.

Just as financial accountants keep track of what goes in and out of the money bank, we calorie accountants will keep track of what goes in and out of the body bank! There are specific tools of the trade you will require to excel in your apprenticeship, first and foremost being your handy-dandy **Loser Ledger**, included in the back of the book.* Much like a checkbook, you will record your tabulations here, keeping a strict daily log of *deposits* (calories in) and *payments* (calories out) and will be able to monitor your account balance regularly. Here's an example:

LOSER LEDGER

Monday	2/12	158	1475
DAY	DATE	WEIGHT	BMR

Time	Food	Cals In	Exercise	Cals Out
8:00	Eggs / Turkey Bacon	202		
10:00			3-mile run	300
12:00	Chicken Caesar Salad	350		
5:00			Walk home from work	100
6:00	Blueberry Soup	83		
7:30	Progresso Lentil Soup	300		
9:00	Handful Cool Whip	58		

| Totals | Add "Cals In" Column → | 993 | Add "Cals Out" Column → | 400 |

$$\boxed{993} - \boxed{400} - \boxed{1475} = \boxed{-822}$$

Calories In   Calories Out   BMR   Total Net Calories

---

* Tree-huggers opting for electronic checking can do so at calorieaccounting.com.

Next, unless you're actually some kind of math whiz, you'll need a **calculator** on hand at all times. (Most cell phones include this application, but if you're living under a rock, I remember having enjoyed my TI-83 in high school.)

Third. Like it or not, you're going to need a **camera**. That's right porky-pine, you're going to be dabbling in the art of self-portraits. Many times we don't even see the fat on our frames until it's confirmed for us photographically, so if you want to stay on top of your goals, you will keep a visual diary of your progress. Just make sure that after you save these photos to a top-secret folder that no one will ever find, your camera has an immediate and reliable function to "Delete Forever." And you'll have no problems!* I know it sucks, but these photos are for your eyes only, and you've got to confront this thing head-on. If you're going to be successful, you have to be honest with yourself. Which brings me to our next tool . . .

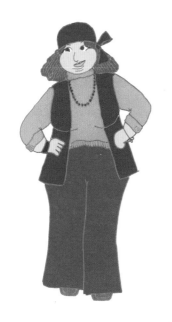

** ***Hippy Hippie Tip!***

Put a bag on it! It's easier to look at blubber when it doesn't have a face. Try taking your selfie with a bag or a nylon or a mask on your head, and you won't identify so personally or emotionally with the plump subject at hand. If this obstruction makes taking the picture impossible, bag it after the fact—try using stickers! Slap 'em on your printed portraits, take yourself out of the situation, and be on your merry way! For extra DIY authenticity, cut and tape a selection from our crafty "Masks" section in the back of the book!

The Scales of Justice. I'm a Libra, so maybe that's why this next component is so important to me. It is certainly true that success on a diet is reflected hugely in the way we feel and the way our clothes fit us, and I'm all for all of that. But in Calorie Accounting, by its very definition, we're playing a numbers game. You will face the scale and weigh yourself before starting anything, and will continue to track your numbers in your Loser Ledger as you make your way. A number is a number and a feeling is a feeling. We will learn to separate the two. But a number is necessary. It's the only way to accurately measure the progress of your program. It will be okay. I promise.

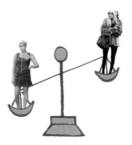

Pedometer. Some of us are telemarketers and some of us are mailmen. Some of us wear commuters to work, some of us never change out of our slippers. We're all different, and we all get a different amount of activity in our day-to-day. But assuming the bulk of us are at least somewhat mobile, we must remember that every step we take is one in the right direction. Keep track of your daily steps to be converted to Calories Out in your Loser Ledger. Especially on days you can't make it to the gym, this little detail's going to be your saving grace.

Optional tool: **Tape measure**. It can be fun to track your loss in inches, and this is certainly a direct correspondent to pounds dropped and lookin' good in general. The Loser Ledger includes a space to track your measurements, where you can record your success. But don't you forego photos and weight in favor of inches. Not the same. Not good enough. These stats are only supplementary. Get it? Got it? Good.

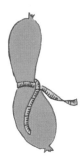

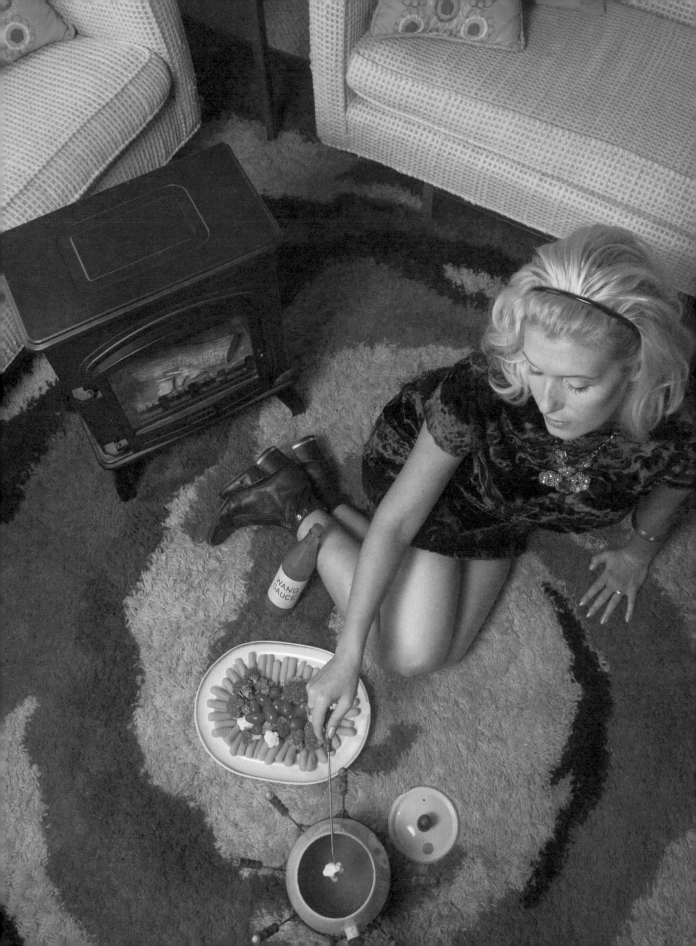

Workbook!

Flash back to math class, someday-skinnies. We're about to build up those calculator calluses all over again.

In order to ensure your full understanding of the glorious Equation of Equations of Equations, and to apply its numerical wonder-workings to your weight loss efforts moving forward, please compute and complete the puzzles below:

1. Martin is a fatty. He has the tits and ass of a Kardashian, but that's a rough road when you're a 32-year-old man. At 5'8" and 255 pounds, he has a BMR of 2,081. Martin is going on vacation to the Cayman Islands with his wife in 5 weeks, but he can't fit into the banana hammock she bought him for Christmas, and she expects him to wear it daily on the beach. Martin estimates that he needs to shed 18 pounds before the hammock can cover his nether-region appropriately. What's his plan of action?

   Martin needs to lose _____ pounds per week.

   Martin needs to net a deficit of _____ calories per week.

   Martin needs to net a deficit of _____ calories per day.

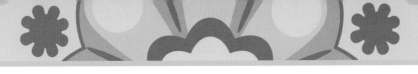

Today, Martin consumed 1,650 calories, and is heading to the gym for his workout. How many miles must he log on the treadmill in order to hit his daily calorie deficit goal? _____

(ANSWERS: 3.6; 12,600; 1,800; 13.69mi)

2. Jenny is a fatty. She has eaten nothing but cheese for the last 3 years and is beginning to resemble a giant wheel of brie. She has BMR of 1,730 and wants to lose 25 pounds. She refuses to work out, but she'd like to aim for the healthy goal of 1.5 pounds lost per week. How many calories should Jenny eat per day, and how long will it take her to lose the 25 pounds on this regimen?

Calories per day _____

How long to goal _____

(A: 980; a little over 4 months)

3. Petunia is a fatty. She goes to the Cici's Pizza Buffet every Friday after work and stays there till they kick her out, or till all the buffalo chicken pizza is gone, whichever comes first. She wants to do a skimpy boudoir photo shoot for her boyfriend, but her love handles are spilling out over her whale tail. She needs to drop 5 pounds in 2 weeks. She is 5'2", 26 years old, and 148 pounds.

What is Petunia's BMR? _____

What is Petunia's deficit goal? _____

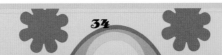

What is her average deficit goal per day? _____

Today, Petunia ate 687 calories. How many calories must she burn with exercise in order to hit her daily goal? _____

(A: 1,468; 17,5000; 1250; 469)

4. Mercutio is a fatty. He works out every day but eats nothing but bagels and drinks nothing but Frappuccinos. He is not willing to change his diet, but he will take in less of it if need be. He will continue to run 5 miles on the treadmill every day. He has a BMR of 1,928.

   If Mercutio eats 1,200 calories worth of bagels and Frappucinos per day, plus keeps up his 5-mile runs, what will his caloric deficit be every week? _____

   At this rate, how much weight will he have lost after 8 weeks? _____

   (A: 8,596; 19.65 lbs)

Who got 100%??? If you passed, give yourself a gold star!!

Keep crunching those numbers, my rotund darlings, and I swear to you, you'll never have to do a crunch again.

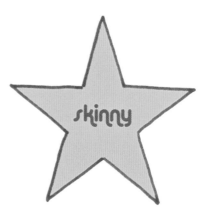

skinny

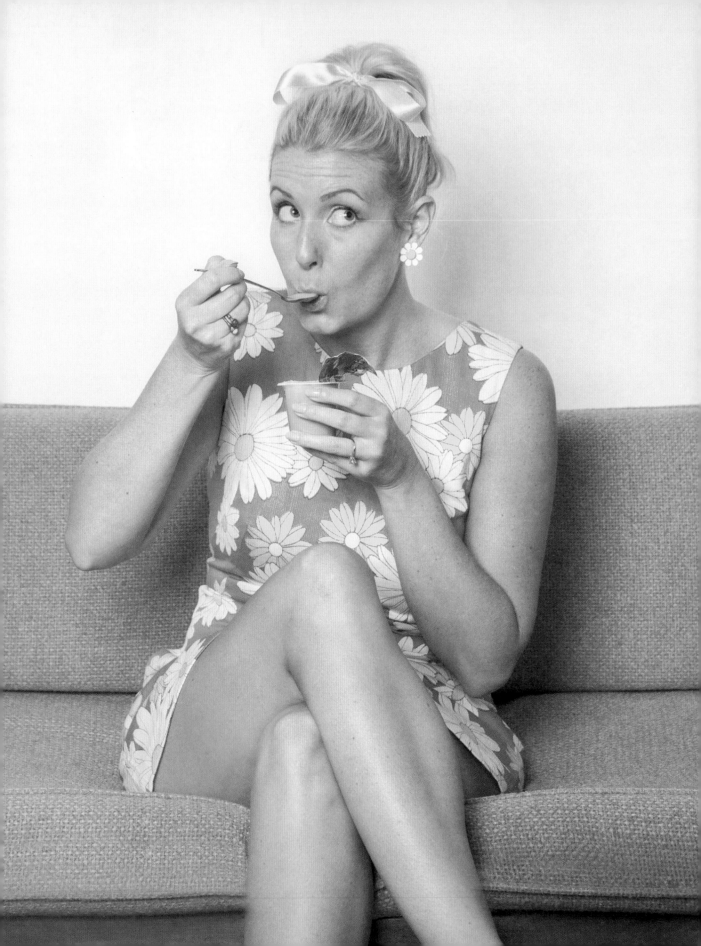

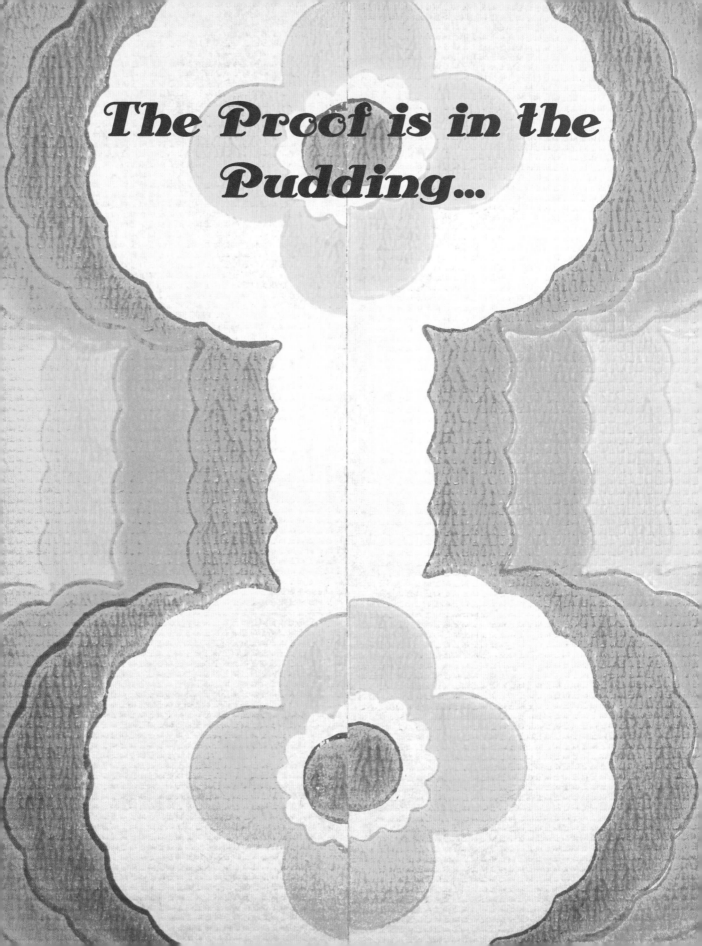

The Proof is in the Pudding...

But Don't Eat the Pudding!

If I am willing to humiliate myself for you, then you should be able to humiliate yourself for you. YOU MUST TAKE PHOTOS, AND YOU MUST LOG THEM! If not here, then in a lockable diary in a safe below your trapdoor.

Here. Look at the tub o' lard I once was:

And then…

Skinny Mofo!

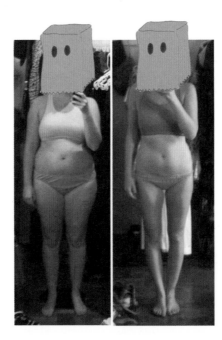

It took a while to get there, but I got there, and I'm glad I've got evidence. You can do it, too!!

A few guidelines for your photojournal:

1. TAKE A STARTING PHOTO! Just do it.
2. Take a new photo each week, at the same time of day, in the same place, from the same angle, wearing the same(ish) thing.**
3. Put a bag or a mask on your head (remember--adorable and plentiful tape-on mask selection in back!) to "remove yourself from the situation."
4. Every week, hold your starting photo next to your newest photo to gaze upon your REAL RESULTS! This is especially useful during plateaus. The scale might be stubborn, but looking back from whence you came can be everything you need to keep from self-destructing (read: ordering 3 pizzas and a side of birthday cake for lunch).

A picture says a thousand words, and the photo-proof is in the photo-pudding.

(If this has made you hungry, go ahead and have a Sugar-Free Snack Pack.)

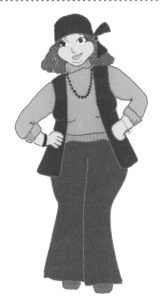

** *Hippy Hippie Tip!*
Behold your behind! Straight-on frontal (not full frontal, gross!) angles are your focus, but if you can negotiate a backside selfie situation, snap away—it'll feel great to monitor a shrinking caboose too!

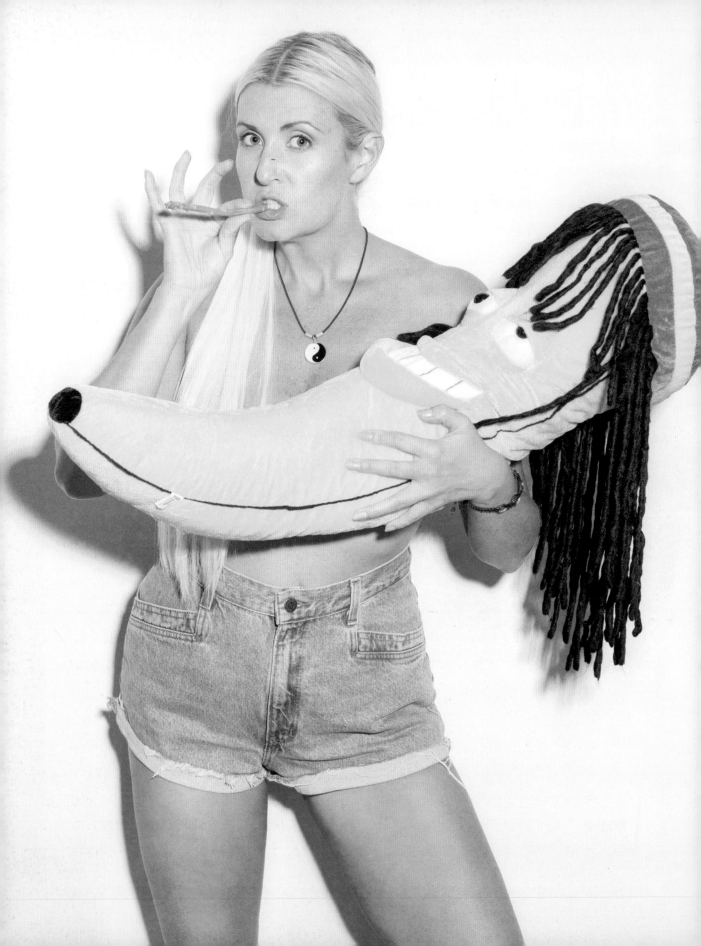

I'm Real

As J. Lo once crooned all Bronxian-sincere-like (with the expert accompaniment of a young Mister Ja Rule), *I'm real*. Well, she's not, she's the farthest thing from it, but she articulates the point I'm hoping to make.

Much as I wish I were, I am not J. Lo. I am not Kate Hudson, I am not Jessica Alba, and I am not an Olsen twin. I have unhealthy obsessions with their unattainable figures, just like every woman does. They're curvy and skinny at once. They're flat and they're busty, depending on whatever looks better with their outfit. They have skinny, sinewy arms and bowed legs with thigh gaps you could stick a donut in between. They have gorgeous collarbones and zero wrinkles, thick hair and white teeth, perfect accessories and no worries. Right? (FYI, it's not like I don't *know* I'm sick in the head.)

If I had their kind of dough, maybe I would hire Harley Pasternak and Tracy Anderson and fucking Hilaria Baldwin to make me toned and healthy and beautiful and forever young. Maybe I would pop in for Botox after a ladies' lunch, or get hooked up to a human growth hormone IV, or spend a month at a lavish New Mexican wellness spa on a liquid cleanse, shitting my brains out, coming away diminutive and positively glowing. But you know what? It's a scam. Even if I did have their money, and even if I did spend it on all the most expensive, luxurious, exclusive health and beauty and fitness products, I still wouldn't look like them. I couldn't. Celebrities are celebrities for a reason. (Besides, like, Kate Gosselin and JWoww). They are striking, special, beautiful beings that are, for the most part, on another level. This doesn't mean they're smart or funny or talented or enjoyable or anything. But the way they look—their bodies, their skin, their faces—this is something inherent for them and impossible for us. Sure they work hard at perfecting and maintaining it, but the starting point is the difference. Some regular schmuck can't just *become* Gwyneth Paltrow. That goop is something you're born with. This is a truth we have to accept, and once we've accepted it, we are free.

All that said, look to me because I am real. I am hardly perfect, I am hardly celebrity-level pretty or skinny or disciplined. And don't get me wrong, I'm plenty confident! But I am supremely regular, and I am attainable. I've lost lots of weight because I worked really hard, but I'll never look perfect in a swimsuit and I can't stop eating cheese. I'm just like you, so you know you can be just like me.

I Luh Ya, Papi.

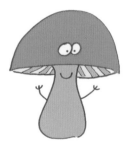

Budgeting Your Bulge Away

It can be assumed that most of the fatties reading this book maintain some semblance of a livelihood, or, at the very least, know how to beg/turn tricks/rob banks and apply their earnings to the sundry and sordid habits they call a life. Whatever pays the bills. Point is, you have bills, and you pay them. And if that's not the case, I don't appreciate you shoplifting my book, the authorities have been notified, and now you'll never get thin.

Budgeting is the most basic component in responsible money management. You look at what you have, you look at what you need, you look at what you want, and you find a way to ration it all out in a system customized specially for you. Same thing in Calorie Accounting. Establish a dream and finance its reality, either penny by penny or calorie by calorie. Here's how.

Step One: Your Starting Balance

Swallow your pride and get up on that scale. You can't settle on a goal without knowing what you've got going for or against you. You might think you'd be happy losing 30 pounds just by assessing your ass in the mirror, but it's not till you weigh in and find out you've actually got a good 50 to drop that you can really budget your plan effectively. (Just playing devil's advocate. From experience.) So come on. Step up. Who cares what the number is—get over it. We are left-brained logical book-keepers now, and we are not distracted by what a number *means*. It just *is*. Record your weight as your Starting Balance in your Loser Ledger. **

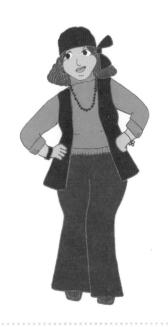

** *Hippy Hippie Tip!*

Be a morning person! Cut yourself a break and weigh yourself in the mornings, when your number will almost always be at its lowest. To put some real spring in your step, try to get a morning workout and/or poop in first! This diet business can be grueling, and the Scales of Justice can be the most annoying part. You deserve to record the numbers when they're at their best.

Step Two: The Goal Mine

Before you give yourself the chance to blubber away about how blubbery you've become, look to the future. The bright, bright, skinny future. You know how much you weigh . . . now how much do you *want* to weigh? Chew over the chart below to target a healthy goal weight for your height.

Female Height to Weight Ratio				Male Height to Weight Ratio			
Height	Low	Target	High	Height	Low	Target	High
4'10"	100	115	131	5'1"	123	134	145
4'11"	101	117	134	5'2"	125	137	148
5'0"	103	120	137	5'3"	127	139	151
5'1"	105	122	140	5'4"	129	142	155
5'2"	108	125	144	5'5"	131	145	159
5'3"	111	128	148	5'6"	133	148	163
5'4"	114	133	152	5'7"	135	151	167
5'5"	117	136	156	5'8"	137	154	171
5'6"	120	140	160	5'9"	139	157	175
5'7"	123	143	164	5'10"	141	160	179
5'8"	126	146	167	5'11"	144	164	183
5'9"	129	150	170	6'0"	147	167	187
5'10"	132	153	173	6'1"	150	171	192
5'11"	135	156	176	6'2"	153	175	197
6'0"	138	159	179	6'3"	157	179	202

Step Three: What Price Skinny?

Now that you know what you want, the question is, can you *afford* it? Well, what's the pensive pause for?! I knew you were big-boned but I never took you for a total dummy! Of course you can afford it! This is America!* You can afford any stretch Hummer or indoor shooting range that liberated mind of yours can dream up! All it takes is a price tag. Then you take a look at your assets, your income, your expenses . . . and from there, all you've got to do is save.

In Calorie Accounting, we'll use our currency—calories—in the exact same way. No matter what the "price tag" for your goal weight may

---

* To be inevitably edited in second print once Calorie Accounting becomes an international phenomenon.

be—20 pounds, 50 pounds, 100 pounds—you'll save up for it just like you would for material treasures. You'll consider your assets (BMR), your income (Calories In), your expenses (Calories Out), and, calorie by calorie, you'll save your way to skinny.

Step Four: The Payment Plan

Before we dig any deeper into caloric budgeting, let me just say this: It is my advice to *not* put yourself on a super-duper time-sensitive diet plan. It's good to set benchmarks and checkpoints and reach for milestones to stay motivated, but if you try to squeeze your system into the confines of time crunches, you're way more apt to make poor investment decisions (i.e. screw up and binge like a mofo). If your goal is to successfully zip up a bridesmaid's dress in two weeks, I would honestly recommend a liquid cleanse. Just know that one bite of wedding cake is going to send you crawling back to me on your hands and knees. So hopefully you have the luxury of a little time on your side. A diet, unstressed, is a doable thing. Now. Knowing what you know about the simple math behind Calorieconomics, let's break up the big picture.

- **Set a weekly budget.** How much weight do you want to lose each week? Keep it healthy, and keep it attainable. One to two pounds a week is typically described as healthy weight loss. In caloric terms, this means a weekly deficit of 3,500 to lose one pound, 7,000 to lose two pounds, etc.
- **One day at a time.** Divide your weekly deficit goal by 7 and there's your daily deficit goal: -500 a day for one pound, -1000 a day for two pounds, etc.

- **BMR in your back pocket.** Remember that this value, your net worth, is always on your side.
- **Know yourself.** What are your strengths and weaknesses when it comes to diet and exercise? Are you someone who likes to snack on mass quantities of anything while sitting in front of the TV for hours (autobiographical), or do you think you could be pretty effective at starving yourself? How good are you about getting to the gym? How much activity is there in your workday? Or your unemploymentday? Are you meaner to the people around you when denied Pop-Tarts or when forced onto the StairMaster? When someone offers you a tossed salad, what's your gut response? Consider all these truths about yourself before you jump into the pit.

Let's draw up an example. Say you're running a BMR of 1,675 and you want to lose two pounds this week. That's going to mean a deficit of 1,000 calories each day. You could eat 675 calories and call it a day (almost assuredly going to bed hungry and homicidal), or you could eat 1,275 calories and get in 600 calories worth of exercise (about six miles on the treadmill—kind of daunting unless there's a *Nanny* marathon on Lifetime), or you could eat 975 calories and burn 300 calories . . . you get the picture. Any combination will do. But an important thing to bear in mind is that a 1,000-calorie deficit per day is really only recommended if you have more than 20 pounds to lose. Less than 20, don't get greedy—that's gotten the better of you these days. Stick to trying to drop a pound a week. Capisce?

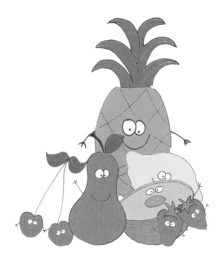

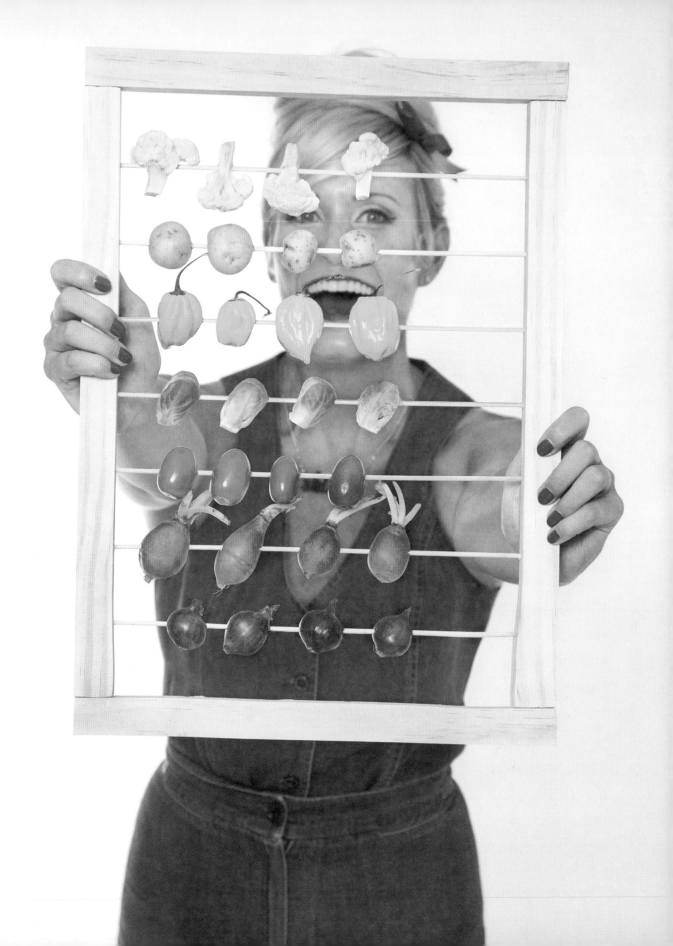

Left Brain Logical

Dear plump-diddly-umptious little reader-friend,

This is the part where I save my own ass, while helping you whittle yours away.

In the world of Calorie Accounting, never forget: we are left-brained logical number crunchers. We live and die by the digits; calories are our only currency; the Equation of Equations of Equations is our bread and butter (don't we wish). All that said, we are also accountable for not being idiotic in our approach. We need to be logical human beings as much as we are logical bookkeepers. I trust that each and every one of you is fully aware that a kale salad is more nutritious than a Mr. Goodbar. But just to make sure all our bases are covered and no one is going to jail for pushing a lifestyle book about surviving on Cool Whip, let's chat.

Because I am a regular gal in a regular world trying regularly to lose weight, I can only assume that there are others out there like me. In my assumption, I'd like to think that those others are just as knowledge-able and experienced as I am; this is not their first diet rodeo, after all. That said, Calorie Accounting is not meant to be a beginner's course in dropping pounds. If not advanced, this is at least intermediate. There are prerequisites in order for one to qualify as a Calorie Accountant, and to maintain that proud title in an intelligent, educated, and healthful way. We must be well-versed and in accordance with the following Level One truths:

1. There is a difference between diet and nutrition. Nutrition is the most important thing in the world—for your health, for your gut, for your muscles, for your eyes, for your skin, for your hair, for your privates, for your longevity, for your everything. Keeping your body active and well fueled with great, gorgeous, natural foods should be, in the long run, everyone's number one priority. Calorie Accountants know this already. And we respect it. It's always in the back of our minds. For now, though, we're just trying to lose the weight. That's the diet part. But that doesn't mean our diet has to be fraught with malnutrition. We are being sensible and logical and taking what we all already know about the imperative virtues of good nutrition, and applying it to this new approach to our weight-loss diets. Yes?

2. There is a difference between a dietician, a nutritionist, and me, some schmuck who lost 35 pounds and can tell you how she did it.

3. Carbs are bad.

4. Sugar is bad.

5. Gluten is bad.

6. Caffeine is bad.

7. Fat is bad.

8. Some fat's not terrible (avocados, nuts, olive oil).

9. Spoiled milk is bad.

10. Anorexia is bad.

11. Bulimia is bad.
12. Addiction to laxatives is bad.
13. Smoking is bad.
14. Drinking is bad.
15. Heroin is bad.
16. Vegetables are good.
17. Lean protein is good.
18. Keeping up with the Kardashians is good.
19. Fiber is good.
20. Vitamins are good.
21. Quinoa is good.
22. Hiking is good.
23. SoulCycle is good.
24. 500 calories worth of Clark Bars is less nutritious than 500 calories worth of arugula.
25. Sleep is good.
26. Mental wellness is good.
27. Pooping is great!

These are the things that we know. The "doy!" factors. The "repeats." The things that have been drilled into our heads so many times we're hardwired to consider them in every decision we make. If you don't know these things, you're officially being held back from advancing into Calorie Accounting. TiVo a month of Dr. Oz and get back to me when you're fully developed.

Love,
Mandykins

Earning Your Meal

"Please, suh. I wan' some mo'."

Sure Oliver, but take a note from Bob Cratchit and put in an honest day's work if you think you deserve to gulp down another bowl of Progresso lentil soup.

Money can't buy happiness, but yes it can. It can buy clothes and jewelry and houses and cars and boob jobs and hand jobs and ice cream. And if you are someone who values these finer things in life, you work hard to earn the money it takes to buy them. Similarly, saved-up calories can absolutely buy happiness. We work hard to earn the caloric cash it takes to stuff our faces with the number one luxury we drool over: food.

In the world of Calorie Accounting, we are fiscally conservative. We prefer not to dabble in the dangerous world of credit accounts, where we buy now, pay later. Instead, we operate from a debit account, where we spend what we've earned, save what we can, and manage real and present cash flow. Put in the work, reap the reward. Earn it.

The feeling of pride and strength and lightness that comes after a three-mile run on the treadmill can be unbelievably satisfying on its own. You catch yourself in the gym mirror, drenched and spent, and think with a smile, "Heck yes, you sexy bitch. Crushin' it!" You might even give yourself a high five in that mirror if no one is looking. But you've got dollar signs in your hungry eyes, and this run just paid you 300 smackers—it's there in your pocket for spending or saving however you like. You've earned it, you're rolling in it, it's disposable income, and that accomplishment high feels amazing. Pay Day! (Want one? You can probably afford it!)

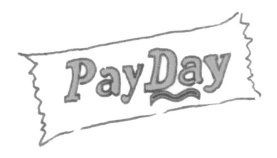

Whether you prefer to treat yourself to a pepperoni slice tonight, pocket the cheddar to pay for bagel day in the office tomorrow, or put it away for the next time your boyfriend brings home Taco Bell, this is your money, and you can do with it what you want. Kate Moss once said, "Nothing tastes as good as skinny feels." While I tend to agree (though I don't have her willpower or her coke habit), I think the more applicable philosophy for Calorie Accountants is: "Nothing tastes as good as a hard-earned meal." Working hard feels good, working hard makes you legitimately hungry, and food tastes best when paired with actual hunger. It all checks out for a very responsible balance.

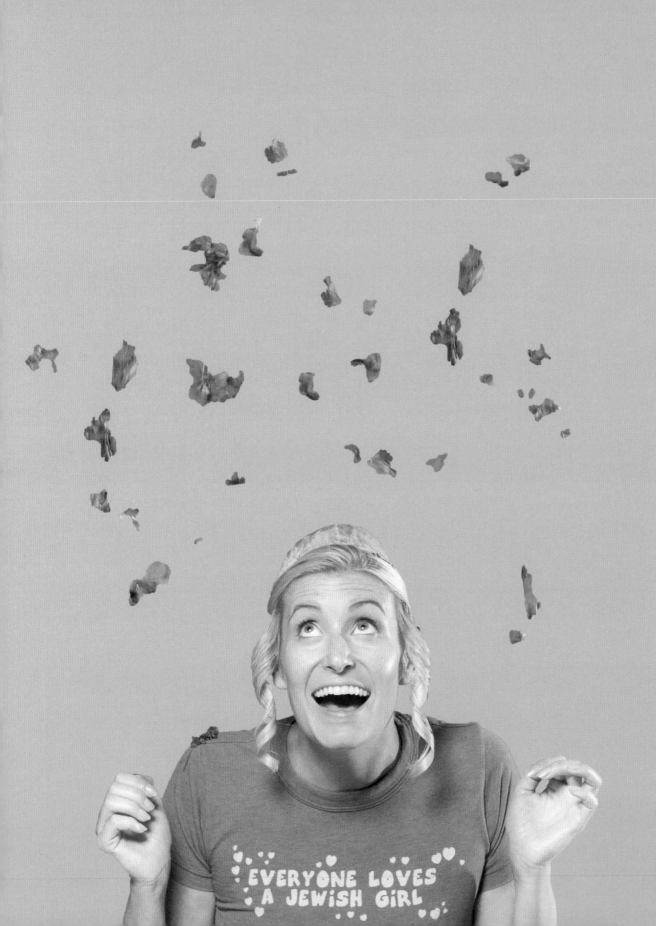

Getting Your Calorie's Worth, or, The Jew in All of Us

Say, Goldenstein!
Yes, Rosenfeld?
What kind of schlemiel are you, paying full price for that gefilte fish!?
What's this you are saying to me, Rosenfeld? You, the putz who missed a BOGO sale on matzo balls?
Oy-yoy-yoy, would you stop with your kibitz and break the challah!?
No noshing for me, bubala, I'm getting svelte.
Calorie Accounting?! Mazel tov!!!!!!!

Now that you know how many calories you have to work with each day to stay within your weekly budget, it's time to stretch those suckers for everything they are. Let's look to my brethren, the Jewish folk, for inspiration. We're famously good with money because we're tight as hell and always looking for a deal. As a result, we've all become rich men. (And women. And womyn.) *Ya ha deedle deedle, bubba bubba deedle deedle dum.* So put on your Jewish hat (if you like, your yarmulke) and learn how to get the most bang for your buck.

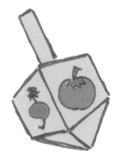

A quick aside

One time I met Joseph Gordon-Levitt. I freaked the fuck out. This is how it went:

MJL: "OHMYGOD!"
JGL: "Hello."
MJL: "HELLO JOSEPH GORDON-LEVITT!"
JGL: "Hello . . ." (motioning for me to complete the sentence)
MJL: (suddenly bashful) "Oh! Mandy!" (coy smile)
JGL: "But what's your full name?"
MJL: "Mandy Jane Levy!"
JGL: "Levy, huh? Then we are descendants of the same Moses!"

And then he bowed, and I curtsied, and we separated.

My mom made me send him an email to ask him to be my boyfriend but he never replied.

Calories add up to pounds just as spare change adds up to dollars. A dollar, or one hundred cents, can be distributed in many ways: 100 pennies, 20 nickels, 10 dimes, 4 quarters . . . and countless combinations thereof. There are just as many ways to distribute your calories. One hundred calories, for instance, can come in the form of a bite-sized Snickers bar. Or it could be half a grapefruit, a quarter cup of Egg Beaters, and a slice of turkey bacon. Or ten bags of mixed greens. Or 50 cherry tomatoes. Or 200 blueberries! Now, Snickers might claim to "satisfy," but if you're asking me, that's only after the whole bag of those bite size turds has made me satisfactorily nauseous. Quarter-Jewess that I am, well, I can't help but go for the better deal. And 200 of most anything is better than one. Am I right or am I right?

Let's Go Shopping!

Did you know that T. J. Maxx stands for Tovah Jacob Makowitz? (I added that to Wikipedia but they took it away.) All I'm trying to say is, my Hebrew homies wrote the book on bargain shopping, and we've got to take a page. Designer duds at discount rates is the name of the game, people. Why buy your Burberry at Bergdorf's when you could get two-for-one and a free reusable tote down the street? Sniffing out those steals may take a little more time and research and focus, but in the end, you can fill your shopping bags without breaking the bank. In *Calorie Accounting*, you'll learn to find the best deals for your diet so you can fill up your plate *and* your tummy while keeping within your budget.

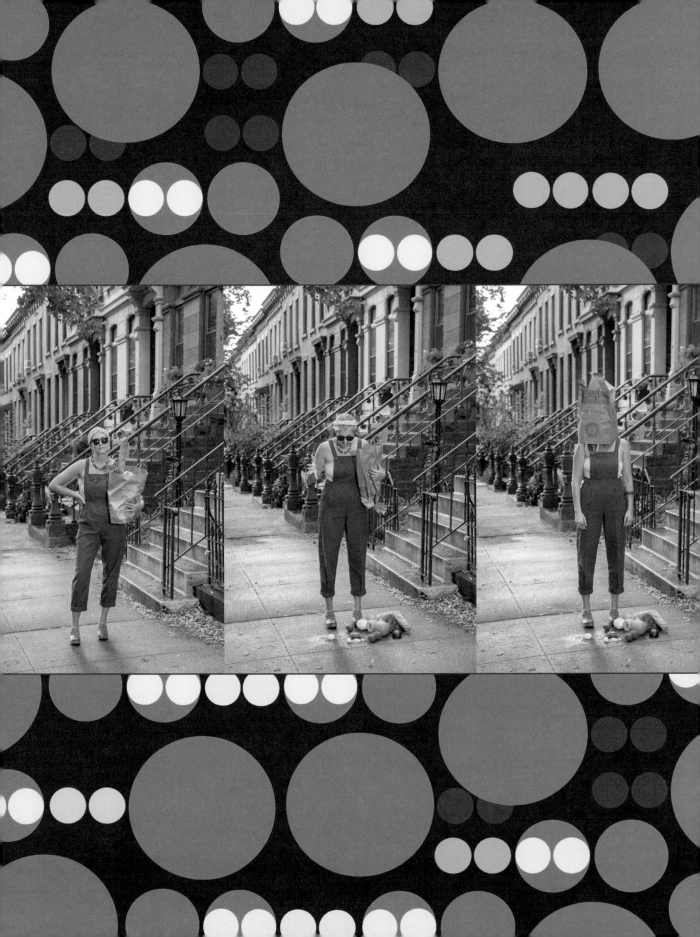

When you're out shopping for clothes, you don't just grab blindly at everything that looks pretty, head straight to the register, swipe the plastic and bounce without blinking an eye. You check out the price tags on the items that intrigue you, try things on, check your bank account, put things on hold, buy things and take them back after using them, etc. It pays to be prudent, after all. Now it's time to do the same thing at the grocery store. Here's how a good Calorie Accountant shops for food as an en*light*ened *consumer* in the *market* place (am I punny or what?!):

1. Nutritionists may urge you in a different direction, but number crunchers don't shy away from **pre-packaged foods.** Why? Because all the facts are there, laid out for you loud and clear. Packaged foods—even packaged produce—have nutrition labels that will provide accurate counts on everything you need to know for your calorie budget. It's a price tag. Now, there's admittedly a lot of gibberish and gooblyguck on these nutrition labels, and most of it is, for what we're doing, worthless. The best part about Calorie Accounting is that the only thing you have to worry about is *calories*, plain and simple. (Well, that and *serving size*. But calories first and foremost.) Not calories from fat, not saturated fat, not daily percentage based on a 2,000 calorie diet, not carbs, not sodium, not sugar, not fiber . . . I mean, it's not going to kill you to *know* about these other components of food and nutrition and the things you're putting into your body, but for all intents and purposes, the bottom line for us is: calories. That's what we're accounting for. So as you browse for packaged food, compare calories on the labels. This can be exciting and fun!

2. Use the **Internet**. For fresh produce from the farmers market and items from the deli or seafood counter, or curious-looking

containers of nuts and berries gathered by your Nepali grocer, no nutritional label will have been slapped on to guide the way. But the Internet is always your friend. Use it. Go to calorieaccounting.com for an expansive database of foods and their nutritional values. Something we don't have? Just google "calories in _____", and you'll find your answer in no time. (Then write to me and let me know what to add to the database! I don't want to make any Icelandic accountant feel left out if I neglected to include sheepsface on the list, after all!)

3. **Time isn't money. Money isn't money. Only calories are money.** When I'm completely devoted to weight loss, this is how I program myself to think: I don't care how many hours or dollars I spend in the supermarket; I will leave no brand of popcorn unturned and will pay no mind to the price per unit; I will make my purchase based solely on how low I can go with my calorie count. I try my best to make out like a bandit in this arena. Regular hot chocolate = 120 calories per package. Sugar free = 70. Fat free = 50. But what's this? *Diet* hot chocolate? On the top shelf? One box left? Twenty-five calories per packet! Booyah! Fifteen bucks a pop!? Whatever! A total steal as far as I'm concerned.[*]

Designer Imposter

OMG you guys, when you're Calorie Accounting, you'll stop being such a label whore and will learn to make some smart substitutions in the marketplace—soon enough, you'll hardly be able to tell the difference!

---

[*] Some readers may be concerned at my lack of concern for traditional "prices" of things, i.e. real money. Look at it this way: if saving calories means you've dried up your bank account, you have no choice but to get skinny the old fashioned way—starvation!

Here are some of the best off-brands to help save you some calories when you've got the urge for expensive taste.

Designer	Imposter
Spaghetti: 1 cup = 220 calories	Spaghetti squash: 1 cup = 42 calories **81% off!**
Mashed potatoes; 1 cup = 237 calories	Mashed cauliflower: 1 cup = 90 calories **63% off!**
Real meat burger = 145 calories	Veggie meat ("chick'n" pattie): = 80 calories **45% off!**
Vanilla ice cream: ½ cup = 137 calories	Fat free Cool Whip: ½ cup = 60 calories **56% off!**
Eggs: 2 = 156 calories	Egg Beaters: 2 equivalent = 60 calories **62% off!**
Milk (2%): 1 cup = 124 calories	Almond milk: 1 cup = 30 calories **76% off!**
Tostitos: 12 chips = 260 calories	Peeled cucumber: 12 pieces = 16 calories **94% off!**
Blueberry pie: 1 slice = 884 calories	Blueberry Soup (recipe on page TK) = 83 calories **91% off!**
Taffy apple: 1 apple = 300 calories	"Taffy Apple" (recipe in back) = 140 calories **54% off!**
Coke = 180 calories	Diet Coke = 0 calories **100% off!**
Rubber	Tofu = 60 calories **70% off!**

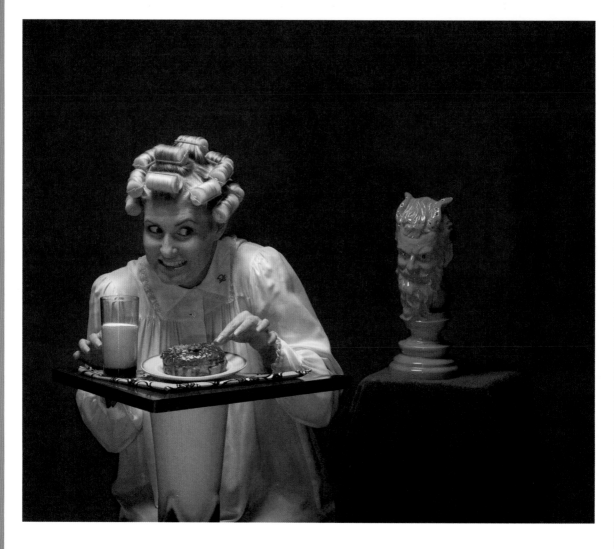

Okay, you know how *People* magazine is always telling us that the way Jennifer Aniston stays fit is a healthy combination of yoga and a balanced diet consisting of things like fish, asparagus, and almonds? Well, my little poopsies, there are certain things (like almonds), which will be the death of you if you're not big on portion control. Jennifer Aniston has about four almonds and says she's full. Normal people can't stop at four. Normal people have 400. And then they gain 400 pounds. You'd be better off, calorically speaking, eating five boxes of Twinkies. (Please don't do that.) So be forewarned and watch your serving sizes. Here are some of the biggest rip-offs in the Calorie Accounting marketplace, healthy and modest as they may appear to the untrained eye:

- Almonds (and nuts in general): 1 oz = 24 nuts = 1 mouthful = **163 calories**
- Avocados/guacamole: 1 fruit = 1 typical serving of guac = **322 calories**
- Olive oil: 1 tbsp = **120 calories**
- Bananas: 1 fruit = **120 calories**
- Cereal: many varieties, but usually 1 cup or less yields **200 calories** or more WITHOUT milk
- Margarine: 1 tbsp = **80 calories**
- Whole wheat bread: 2 slices = **140 calories**
- Cheese: 1 cube = **80 calories** (When's the last time you stopped at one cube at a cocktail party?)
- Chocolate: 1 Hershey's Kiss = **25 calories**. (How fast can you scarf down a bag?)
- Yogurt: around **100 calories**
- Juice: 8 oz orange juice = **120 calories** (My advice is to *eat* your calories, not drink them.)
- Peanut Butter: 1 tbsp = **100 calories**

These Are a Few of My Favorite Things

Like I said, I'm a real cheapskate when it comes to my calorie allowance. I'm also a pretty compulsive snacker. Definitely more of a "ludicrous amount of small meals" gal than a "three square meals" gal. For the mass quantities of food I like to be constantly shoving down my maw while watching basic cable, I really have to find the lowest-calorie options to compensate for this . . . condition.

- Pumpkin seeds: **280 calories** per bag, which is about one sitcom worth of mindless grazing.
- Grape tomatoes: **2 calories** per tomato! I could eat 200 of these a day and I'm hardly joking.
- 100-calorie kettle corn: **100 calories**, duh. Sometimes this can make me bloat, though. FYI.
- I Can't Believe It's Not Butter spray: **0 calories,** bitches! Who sprays? I pour!
- 100-calorie kettle corn drenched in 0-calorie I Can't Believe It's Not Butter spray: **100 calories** of Happiness.
- Fat-free-sugar-free-zero-calorie U-Bet chocolate syrup (tastes like poison alone but works well enough as a dipping sauce for strawberries): **4 calories**/fruit
- Fat free feta cheese: **35 calories**/serving. Does the trick, consistency-wise, on salads. Wouldn't eat it alone.
- Lite string cheese: **60 calories**/stick. Good for snacking on its own, or also for melting on veggie burgers or shredding on salads.
- Tribe eggplant hummus: **35 calories**/serving. All the other flavors are 50.
- Diet Swiss Miss hot chocolate: **25 calories**/pack. Gets your chocolate fix in, and warm things are satisfying.
- Newman's Own Lite Honey Mustard salad dressing – **35 calories**/tbsp, and this serving size is enough. I do take this with me out to eat. Don't roll your eyes at me; I'm thin.
- Bushels upon bushels of blueberries: **83 calories**/cup, which is quite a hefty helping of berries. Enjoy, but make sure there's a toilet nearby.

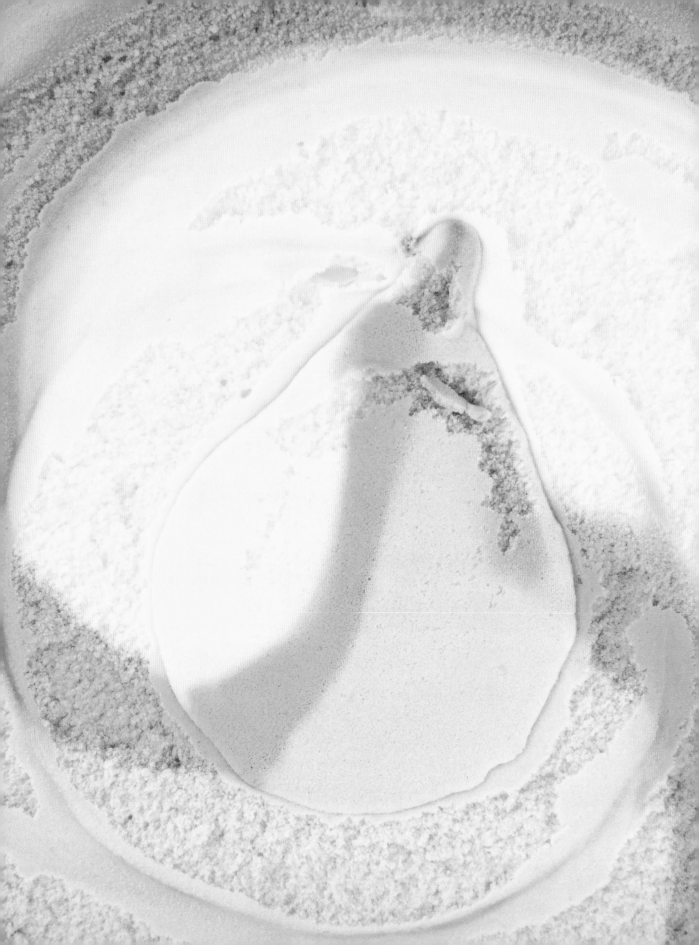

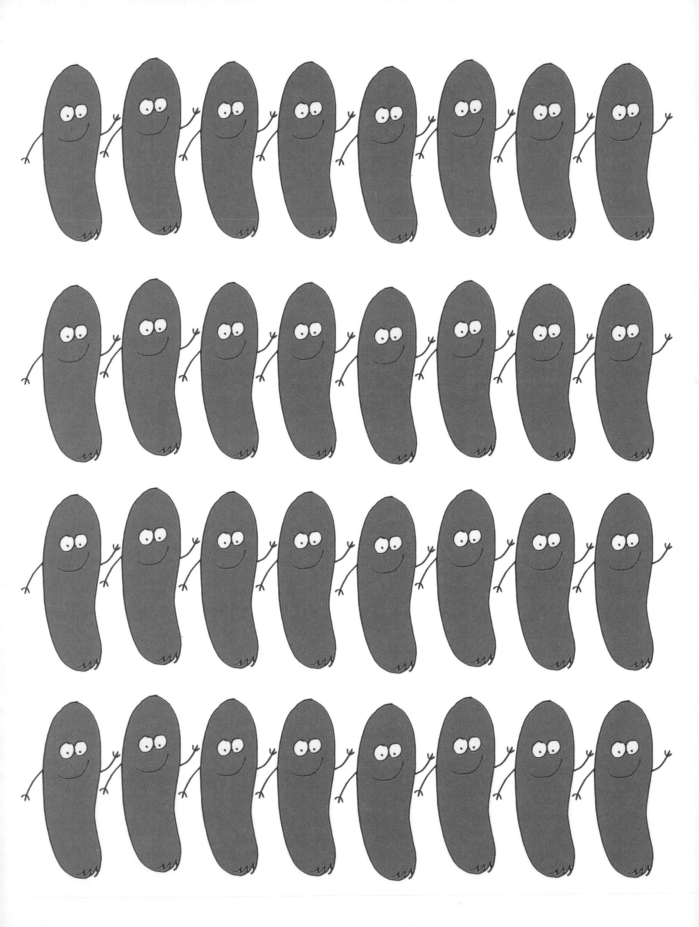

Pickles!!!

When my little sister and I were four and eight, respectively, we used to wake up on weekends at 6:00 a.m. and meet in the family room with wine glasses and a jar of Claussen dills. Without a word, we'd polish off the two dozen spears, until only that big, glorious jug of swishing pickle juice remained. We'd pour the salty, chartreuse libation into each of our glasses, clink to toast the day, then guzzle down the whole jar. And our mother wondered why we had such horseshit breath in the mornings.

I'm so glad my lust for pickles has stayed with me through adulthood. I have found, over my many years of being hungry for one reason or another, that nothing settles a rumbling stomach quite like the crunch of a fresh dill pickle. That salty, vinegary sting will satisfy your hunger more immediately than any fruit, nut, or granola bar. And guess what? Only 5 calories a spear. A freaking steal!!!

If you live in Portland or Brooklyn, you may have easy access to other pickled things, like cauliflower, or green beans, or positive vibes captured in a mason jar. Any old pickled thing can scratch a hungry itch, and as long as you're staying away from the pickled pigs feet (and good god, I hope you are), it won't cost you but a nickel.

Skinny Snax!

Oodles of Noodles

For as long as I can remember, I've had three recurring dreams. In one I'm a pipsqueak on a junior high basketball court, getting schooled and trampled by all the pretty, sporty girls with grosgrain ribbons in their long ponytails, and then suddenly I start flapping my arms (like a freak) and I begin to levitate . . . I flap a little harder and rise a little higher, hovering over the game below, and then my teammate passes me the ball and I fly over to the hoop and SLAM DUNK THAT FUNK, winning the game. The crowd goes wild, and then I fly out of the gymnasium and soar contentedly over my suburban hometown.[*]

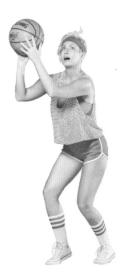

---

[*] While this particular basketball vignette has returned most frequently throughout my life, it should be noted that just casual flying in general is a heavily represented motif in my REM cycle. I've heard it symbolizes a delusional ego.

In another one I'm spooning with Brandon Flowers of The Killers (I'm the big spoon), and when he turns to face me he has some pretty serious T-zone acne, and I'm like, *That's a shame*, and then he's like, "You're not my wife!" and he runs out. Then I take a guitar and start writing a song, and nine times out of ten I wake myself up at this point, breaking through sleep paralysis to actually sing the ditty I've composed. Then I'll grab my iPhone to groggily record the melody, because one of these days I'm going to dream up the next "Yesterday."

And in the last one I'm sobbing tears of happiness, as joyful and ecstatic as I've ever been, stars and hearts and rainbows are dancing around my head. I'm lighter than air, bursting with love and hope . . . and it's all because I'm swimming through a regulation-sized lap pool filled with buttered noodles.

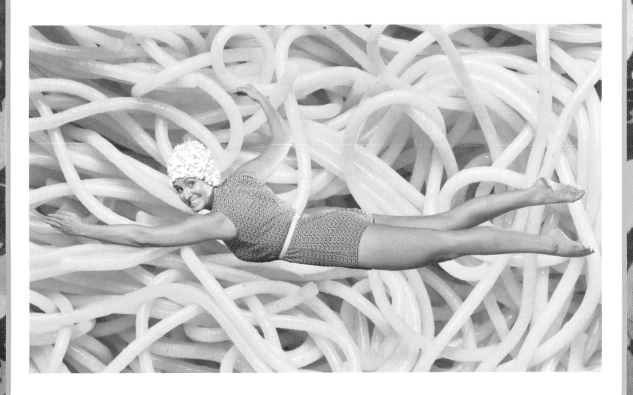

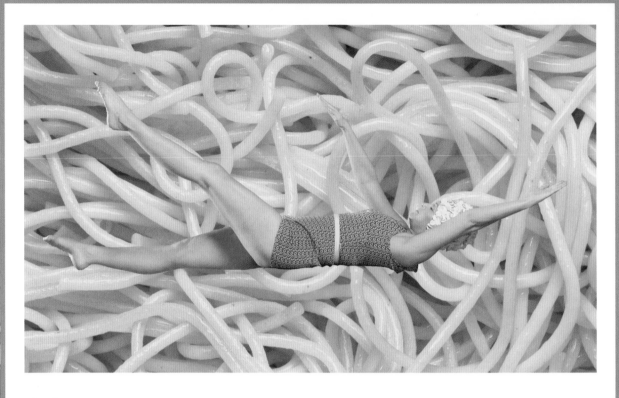

Sigh.

Fat-tastic friends, I know you feel me: Ain't nothin' better on God's green Earth than slurpin' up a big ol' bowl of pasta. Or swimming in one. And quite likely, this taste sensation is precisely why you're here with me now. Carbs are the devil; they've supersized us. And carbs are all of the best things. Carbs are the dough for your pizza, the tortilla for your burrito, the bagel for your schmear. They're cereal, they're mashed potatoes, they're freaking sushi. But can we all agree that when we've tried and failed at the Atkins diet, the hardest carb to cut out was pasta? Olive Garden is the dead end for so many of life's best-laid plans, and this is no exception. But, doughy darlings, if you're like me and feel that life's just not worth living if you can't shove oodles of noodles down your gullet whenever the urge might emerge, then chew on this: shirataki.

I've got your miracle, and it comes from Japan (as all miracles do). Shirataki are thin, translucent, gelatinous, traditional Japanese noodles that are zero fat, zero carb, zero gluten, zero sugar, zero cholesterol, ZERO CALORIE NOODLES.* Not even kidding. I'm sure that they've been placed on this Earth (and in Whole Foods and Asian supermarkets) by Satan himself, and this has been confirmed via a recent Wikipedia session wherein I learned that shirataki are made from "devil's tongue yam." Don't ask, just slurp. We said we'd do anything to get skinny, right?

So here's the thing: don't kid yourself into thinking you can dump a jar of red gravy on these things and you'll be magically whisked away to grandma's Sunday dinner. They're Asian noodles; they're squirmy and weird, they sort of dissolve on your tongue, and frankly they're a little stinky. They're not al dente; they're a means to an end. But for me, and I think for you, too, if I can dupe myself into thinking I'm eating pasta in any capacity and will still be able to lose weight, I'm thrilled.

So think about the pasta that made you fat. Mine was spaghetti with butter and hot sauce and Parmesan cheese. (A box of spaghetti with a stick of butter and a bottle of hot sauce and a jar of Parmesan cheese.) My shirataki fake-out? Shirataki spaghetti (0 Cal), I Can't Believe It's Not Butter Spray (0 Cal), Louisiana Hot Sauce (0 Cal), and 1 tbsp of grated Parmesan (30 cal). ARE YOU KIDDING ME?????? I can have Mandy's Famous Spaghetti Slop for 30 calories per bowl???? Hell, throw a few more tablespoons of cheese on there; I can certainly afford it!!!

---

* If you're a patriot, you can also go for the American-made tofu shirataki noodles. These ones—which come in fettuccine, spaghetti, macaroni, and angel hair—have 10 calories per serving, are a bit more durable, slightly less stinky, and, as I've found, are somewhat "squeaky" in terms of their chewing experience.

Was your noodle offender mac 'n' cheese? You can get shirataki in macaroni form, too, maybe melt some ICBINB spray and fat-free cheddar on top? It might taste like rubber, but it might not! Experiment!

Alternately, make yourself a healthy, sustainable, nutrient-rich shirataki dish! Toss some shirataki angel hair with grilled chicken and veggies, or mix it up with a stir-fry using the shirataki rice. (Or, if you're me, substitute your regular brown rice-with-A.1.-and-Parmesan habit for the shirataki surrogate, and you're golden!)

It all seems too good to be true, and hey, maybe this will be pulled from the shelves tomorrow. But if we're accounting only for calories as numbers and not their nutritional makeup and integrity, I'd say we've got something pretty miraculous here. Slurp up! (But plug your nose.)

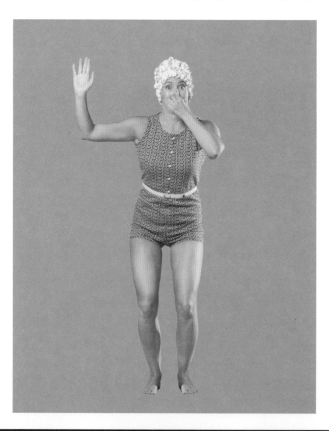

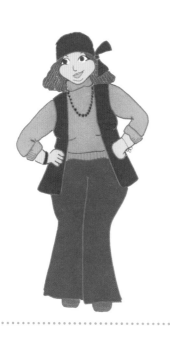

** *Hippy Hippie Tip!*

I know you like to think that your shit don't stank, but your shirataki most definitely DO stank. Stankonia 2000. If you can't stomach the smell, tofu shirataki noodles are a great substitute! These babies, made from tofu AND the devil yam, pack just 10 calories per serving and are a little less nasally offensive. They're still not roses, but they're an improvement.

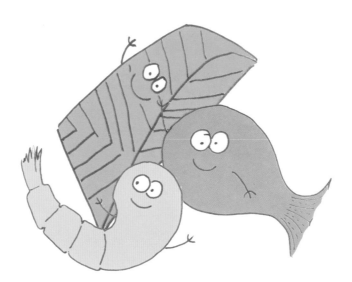

Moving Your Moneymaker

Raise your hand if you hate the gym! Okay, an overwhelming number of books just fell to the floor. Listen. I am a lazy sack of chocolate chip cookie dough at heart like all the rest of you, but at the risk of sounding overly peppy, if you want to change your life, you have to change your attitude. Working out doesn't have to be the bane of your existence, I swear. Calorie Accounting can help.

We rattle off all sorts of excuses why we can't make it to the gym. We're too tired, we have no time, "work's crazy" (spoken with a limp wrist and a fluttering of the eyelids), our grandma died, it's allergy season, our foot hurts, blah blah blah. And the reason we make these excuses is because the gym seems like total bullshit to us! We lift and squat and stretch and sweat but we have no way of tracking how this is really affecting our weight loss goals. So it's just misery and guesswork with no tangible payoff, unless you're chill and patient enough to cross your fingers for six weeks and just hope you'll see results . . . but even then you might find that your waifish tween of a personal trainer has made you run stadiums and consider suicide in exchange for muscle ON TOP OF fat, and suddenly you've got a closet full of dresses with sleeves that won't fit over your bulging man arms! Presumably.

I have a distinct memory of a *Muppet Babies* episode where all the characters have some sort of revolting slop set down in front of them for mealtime, but in order to ingest it with a smile, they all decide to pretend the slop is a heaping ice cream sundae or a seven-layer cake or a mountain of candy. Similarly, in *Hook*, everyone's favorite reinvention of everyone's favorite fairy tale, all the Lost Boys use their power of imagination to make their mess-hall slop fun as well, turning it into a loving

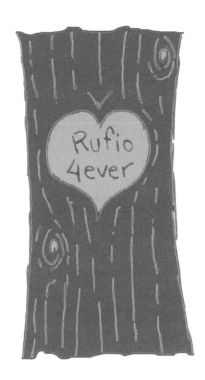

and colorful paintball food fight! Remember? Remember Rufio? Was that John Leguizamo?

Anyway. The point is, sometimes playing mind games with ourselves is the best way to get over an obstacle. Just as the Muppets and Lost Boys love ice cream and paintball, we Calorie Accountants love money! So stop thinking of the gym as your own personal hell, and use your imagination to pretend the gym is the most fabulous and generous purveyor of usable currencies . . . **The Bank!**

Go to The Bank as often as you can. I say daily. I say morning-ly. You go to The Bank to take out a little extra spending money for the day ahead of you. Check it off your list like any other errand and get on with your life, now knowing exactly how many calories you have to spend that day. Endorphins aren't what make you feel happy after working out. It's the cash in your pocket!

Machines Are Our Friends

I struggle with my acceptance of any gym activity that I can't put a price on, i.e. exactly how many calories this is burning for me. I know it's good to lift weights and do crunches and look like a fool with a medicine ball, but if there's not a computer reassuring me that every move I make is absolutely good for something TODAY, then I say forget it. So I stick to aerobic machines. I can adjust levels and inclines and times to correspond with how motivated or unmotivated I'm feeling that day, but the important part is, this is mostly mindless work that enables me to watch TV, the incentive behind pretty much everything I do in life.**

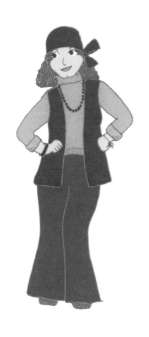

** *Hippy Hippie Tip!*

Don't tell her I told you, but Mandy has a bad attitude and is averse to change! If you love more liberating exercises like golf and tennis and Zumba and yoga and Tae Bo and pogo sticking, please ignore her machine-centric manifesto and keep up your own good work—you can track and account for these burn sessions, too! A wearable heart rate monitor/calorie counter is great but can be a little pricey. To estimate your burn on the cheap, just check online at calorieaccounting.com for numbers on all sorts of alternative exercise, from fencing to gettin' it on!

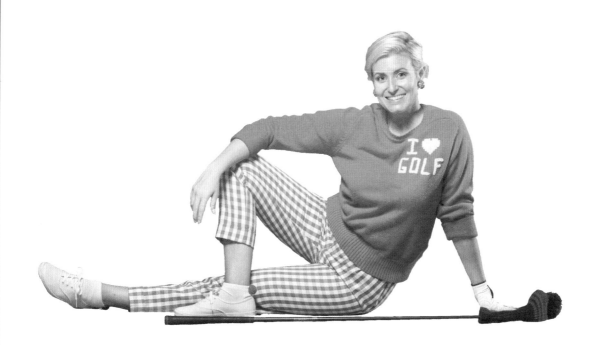

My machine of choice is the treadmill. I base my preference on the fact that the workout it creates is most closely linked to what we humans—nomads at our basest core—are meant to do naturally. My endurance is sometimes frightening. If I didn't have to go to work, I could easily and happily spend all day just walking leisurely on a treadmill, flipping through E! and Bravo and Lifetime. Oh that's another thing—if you already have cable TV at home, you might consider discontinuing your service while you're dieting, and picking a gym based on the channels it offers. Nothing like a *Real Housewives* marathon to motivate your cardio for the day.

I face the treadmill every morning and put no pressure on myself to do anything other than walk. But sometimes I surprise myself, and up the ante to jog a little here and there, and sometimes, for no feasible reason at all, I have the strength and willingness to actually RUN on the treadmill . . . sometimes for miles at a time! I don't know where the energy suddenly comes from, but when it shows its face, I don't thumb my nose. No matter how fast or slow I'm clocking the miles, though, the idea is just that I'm clocking them. **One mile is about 100 calories,** whether you stroll, crawl, skip, crab walk, or sprint the distance. So if you don't want to break a sweat and have all the time in the world, just walk. For however long and however far you want to. And if you have twenty minutes flat to get in a decent workout before hitting the showers and meeting the girls for happy hour, see if you can run it. Same principles go for elliptical machines, bicycles, stairs . . . these all have computers that will tell you how many calories you've burned in your workout. And however many you can squeeze out in a session is just going to add to the riches of your BMR, and, in turn, the total amount of Calories In you can budget for your day! Yes? Get it? The Bank? Money? Fun! Okay!

One other way to really pinch your caloric pennies is to carry around a **pedometer.** Find one for $15 or $20 on Amazon. You may think it's dorky, but when it's the difference between a growling stomach and a Sugar Free Snack Pack at night, you'll thank me. A good Calorie Accountant lets no exchange slip through the cracks. And in addition to our burnings (b*earn*ings?) from The Bank and our daily BMR—which, again, is available to us even if we're developing bedsores—we take many a step in our day-to-day. This extra effort is not to be ignored! Whether you're like me—a sales schmuck schlepping around New York City for hours and blocks and miles at a time—or like me five years ago—a junk mail copywriter who walked from house to car to desk and back each day—you're always doing *something*, and the calories need to be accounted for! And just knowing that you're essentially making money with every step you take can be your motivation to take the stairs or walk to work. So just put your pedometer in your pocket and record your b*earn*ings (Do you hate that? Should I stop that?) at the end of the day. It can be your little bonus to pay for one more late night snack during the Jimmys.

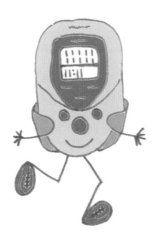

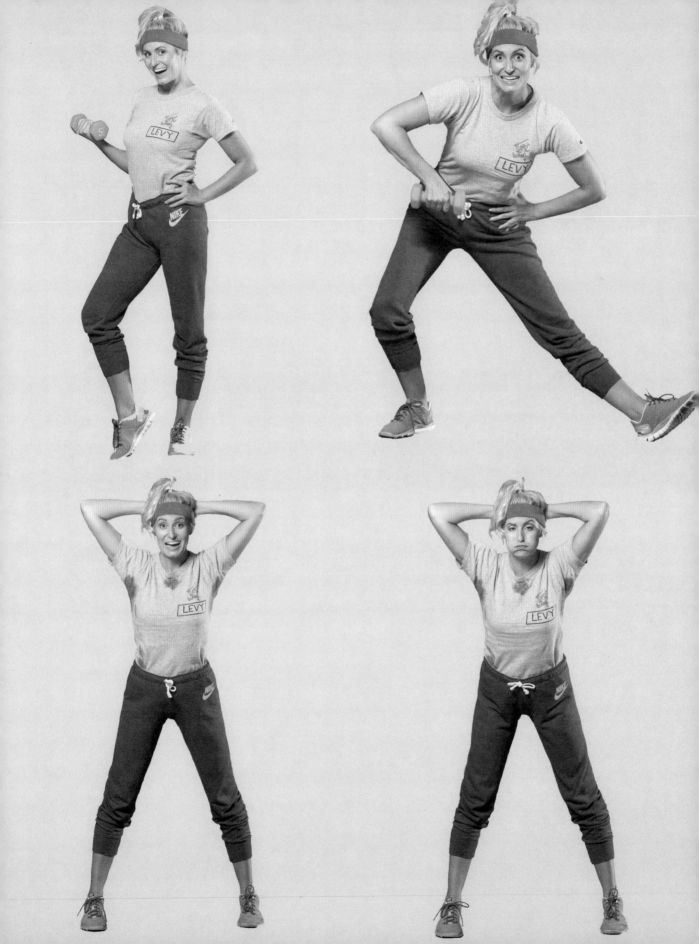

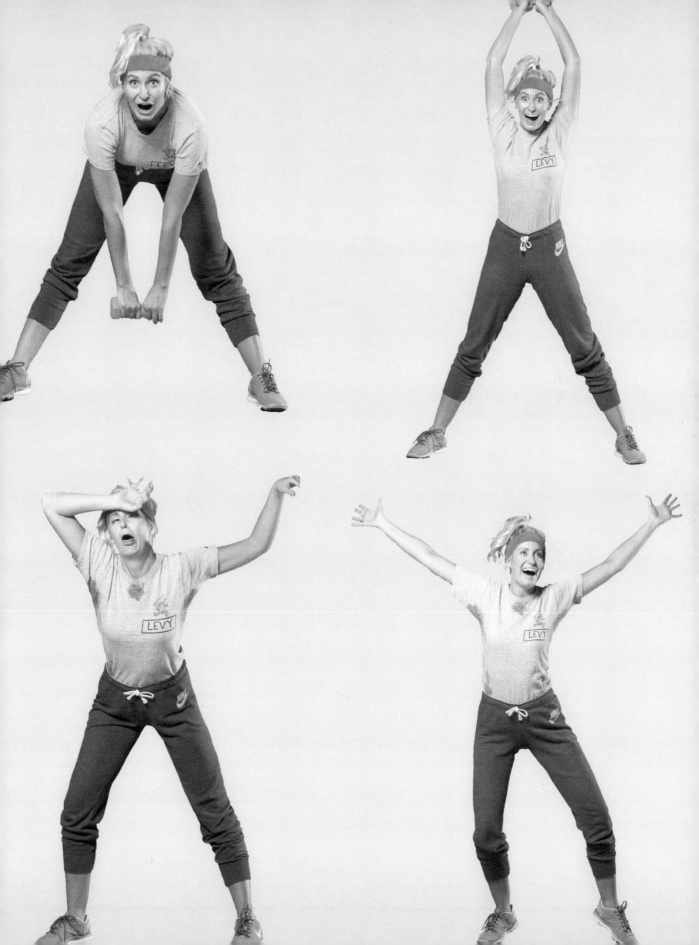

Working for the Weekend

Going away for the weekend? Do yourself a favor and have a blast! How can that possibly be a reality when you're on a diet, and legitimate blasts come only in the form of unrestricted food and drink? Work hard to play hard, round darlings. Here's the occasional strategy for the occasional getaway from your daily Calorie Accounting regimen.

Plan ahead. What's your end game here, to start? Maybe you can't expect to keep losing while you're away, but will you be happy enough with just not *gaining* any weight on vacation? That's a healthy and realistic-enough approach. Calculate your BMR, multiply it by the number of days you'll be off-program, and arrive at the maximum number of calories you can net without getting fat again. (And please, I'm trusting we all know that gaining three or four pounds on vacation is not truly "getting fat again." If it happens, it's easily erasable temporary bloat; I'm just trying to make a point here people.) So for example's sake, say your BMR is 1,500. And say you're going to Atlantic City for a three-day weekend. Net 4,500 calories for your time away and you'll head back home the exact same person as when you arrived. (Unless you contracted genital warts or lockjaw . . . be careful on that boardwalk!)

Know what I'd do?

I'd commit like a motherfucker. I'd put in overtime. I'd take a working lunch. I'd sign up for a night shift. I'd scrimp and I'd save. An extra mile on the treadmill every day, no snacks after dinner, no cheese on my salad, whatever it takes. If there's a light at the end of a misery tunnel, I'll put my head down and power through. For a good week leading up to my vacation, I'd do everything I could to arrive on that first day with all sorts of extra spending loot in my caloric pocketbook. Then I can add my hard-earned deficit to my 4,500, and I've got bonus calories to play with while I'm away! It's like the ten free gambling dollars the casino gives you when you sign up for their rewards card! And those extra bucks can get swallowed up as quickly as three pulls of the slot or three hairs of the dog, but either way, you're glad you were able to account for them. So go ahead, get down with that saltwater taffy. You worked hard for it, you deserve it, and you're a winner!!!

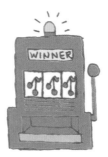

Artsy Fartsy

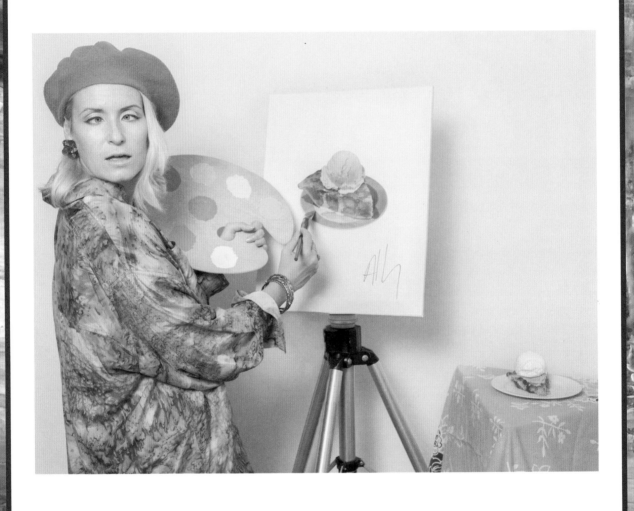

A Calorie Accounting haiku:

Piggy at the trough:
Feasts; Oinks; I identify.
But he can't do math.

A Calorie Accounting limerick:

There once was a fatty named Mandy
Who loved to eat all kinds of candy.
From Snickers to Mounds,
Soon she'd gained forty pounds,
But with Cal. Accounting she's a dandy!

A Calorie Accounting acrostic poem:

So many bitches
Keep up with the Kardashians
I mean, as far as looks go.
No way will I ever be as hot as a SoCal Armenian;
Nevertheless, I'm looking good for a regular schmuck . . .
Yippee!!!!!!

A Calorie Accounting concrete poem:

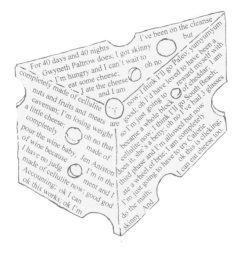

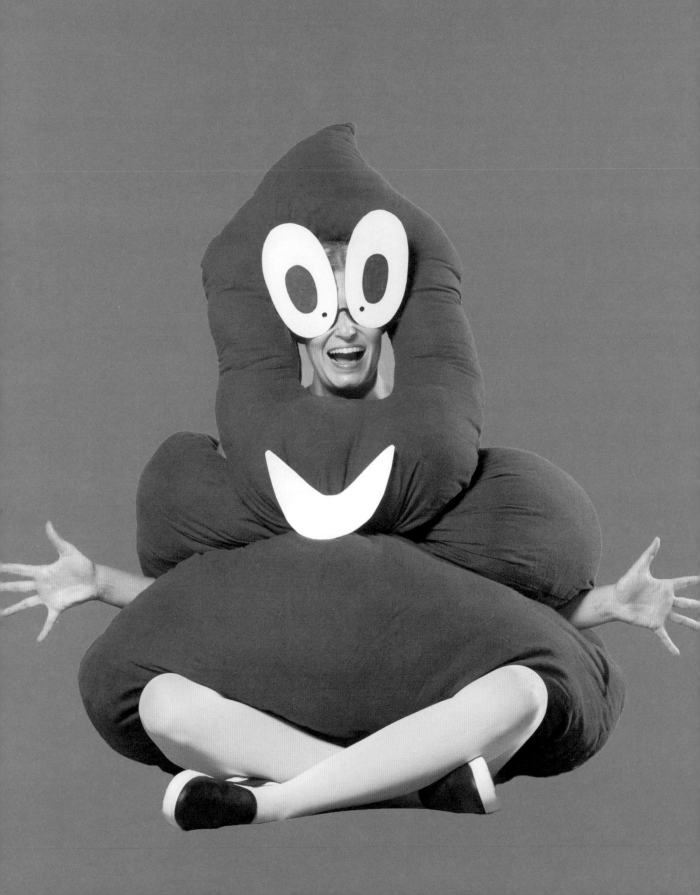

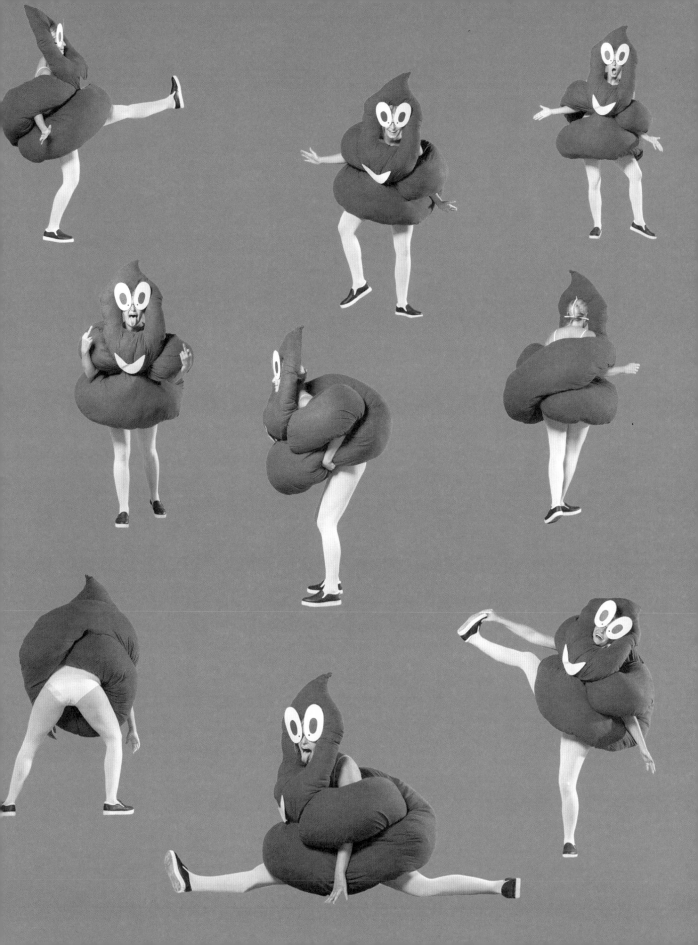

POOP!

I am a senior citizen in so many ways, you guys. When left to my own devices, I watch nonstop *Judge Judy*, I get down to John Denver, I go to the matinee show and complain about the price, I hike my elastic waist pants up to my tits, I spend hours on end in the bingo hall and at the penny slots, and I eat massive amounts of (sugar-free) pudding and Jell-O. And just like a senior, there's nothing in this world that makes me happier than executing a freaking fantabulous B.M.

Poop, poop, poop, I looooove to poop!

Now, don't turn on me, dear readers. I am not a sick weird freak. This is not TMI. I just want us to be able to be real with one another, you know? And everybody poops, and the people who can talk freely about this very beautiful and natural part of life are the people who will find the most satisfaction and success in its magic. You dig? Super! (Pooper!) Now take this into the can and let's chat.

Pooping is always wonderful, but especially when you're trying to lose a few. A good poop feels so healthy, expelling all that poison and junk, leaving you feeling so light and refreshed, so energized and ready to take on the day. Amiright? Your world is a sunnier one all around if you've had a good poop. However . . .

The days without poop are dark and brooding. They are heavy, they are sad. They are made of bloat, and of exertion, and of failure. When the days without poop compound, we feel helpless and ever-expanding . . . how *does* your large intestine accommodate that footlong Spicy Italian anyway???

Stay posi, and stay regular, former fatties. A daily deuce will keep you feeling your best and maintaining your focus. A little stopped up? Here are some pointers and best practices for keeping everything moving smoothly:

1. Eat plenty o' greens. Fresh kale, spinach, arugula, mint. In a salad, in a green juice, via syringe, whatever it takes. These aren't going to add very many C's to your ledger and you know they're the best things for you—gobble 'em down and get on the pot!

2. Drink lots of water! It's like Liquid-Plumr (who knew that was spelled so stupidly?). Hydrate and flush out that clog!

3. Coffee. Strong and black. Watch it go right through you.

4. Prune juice. One time, I went to Japan for two weeks and was full-on constipated the entire time. The amount of live sea urchins and raw quail eggs that were swimming in my stomach for a fortnight was enough to drive me mad, and trolling for MiraLAX in Harajuku only elicited nervous giggles from cosplay shopgirls. I prayed for a poop at every temple, employed the bidet at every ryokan, and drank quantities of Kirin that should make most anyone shit his pants, but nary a gurgle or prairie dog peeked out. Then suddenly, at a rare American breakfast stop

(I was growing tired of young yellowfin with my OJ), I saw it, gleaming in all its splendor, a beacon of hope and relief: prune juice. I drank two 8 oz glasses and was on the toilet in less than five minutes. It was spectacular.

5. Blueberries en masse! A bushel of these and splat goes the doodie.

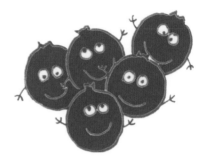

6. Do your squats! Think about this: humans were made so that we could bend our knees, get down low, and poop into holes in the ground. Either dig a hole in your backyard for those hard-to-go days, or do some squatting exercises in your bathroom until you feel things moving. You can also hold your knees to your chest while you're on the pot (but that seems dangerous, like something could rip), or situate your wastebasket in front of the throne, propping your feet and knees up like a real queen. Something will drop!

7. Run for the runs! Another way to get things moving is literally to get moving. Burn calories *and* lighten your load with a quick run around the block.

8. Go to the library. Every time I step foot in a biography section, I gotta take a dump.

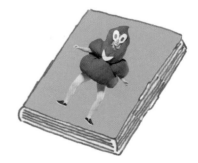

9. Shots! Shots! Shots! Shots Shots Shots! Of olive oil! This can be highly caloric, so make sure you can afford it. But it's an effective constipation-relieving nightcap. Take down a tablespoon or two of extra virgin olive oil before bed, and in the morning, you'll be lubricated and rejuvenated.

10. Swiss Kriss Herbal Laxatives. These are all natural, made of crushed flowers and sunshine. Take a couple one or two times a day, and very manageable, very satisfying poops will follow in about six to eight hours.

Okay, I'm pooped.

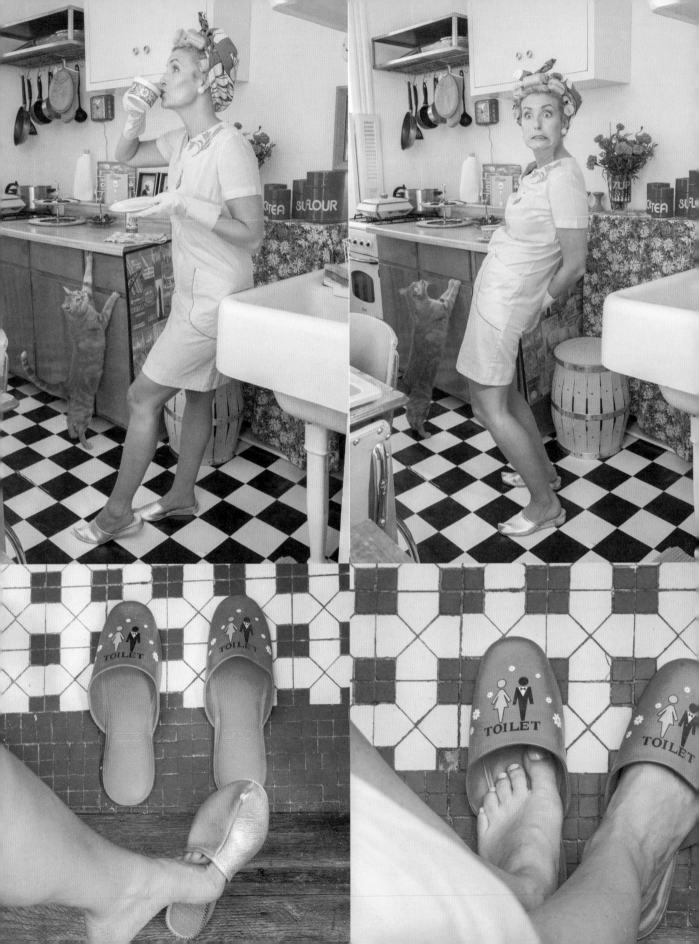

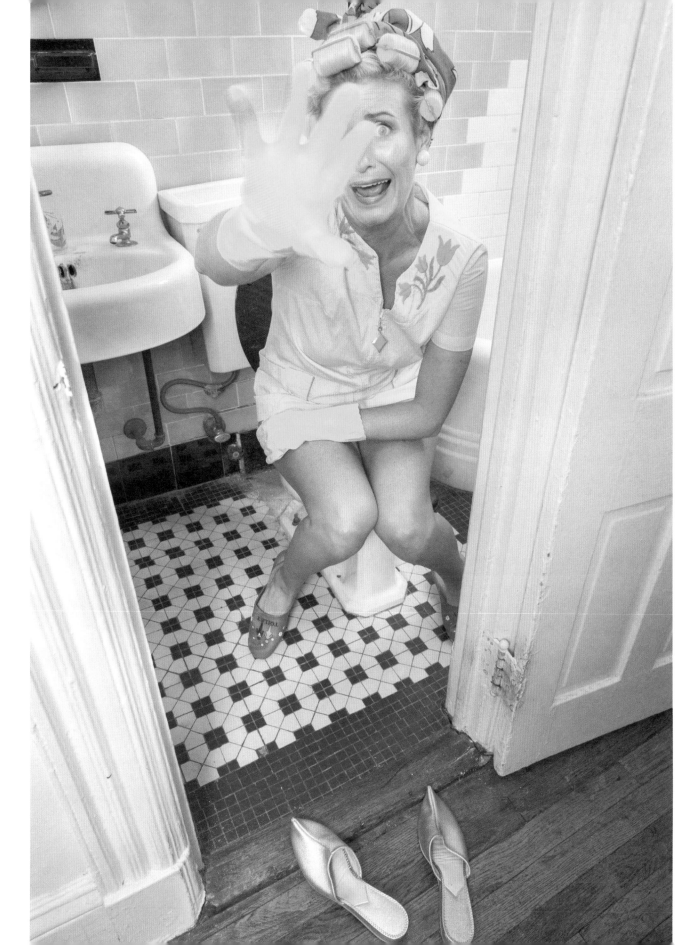

Your Money's No Good Here

If *Pretty Woman* revealed any secrets to the world other than Julia Roberts's chronic struggle with flat footedness and her subsequent inability to streetwalk without looking like she's got a pole up her ass (Sorry! Obviously I love her; she's America's Sweetheart! But girl can be awkward.), it was the simple truth that all a down-on-her-luck gal must do in order to afford an off-the-runway wardrobe is to sleep with Richard Gere. Well. It's a myth. I've tried that. Doesn't work. Snooty Rodeo Drive shopkeepers can smell the poor from miles away. If you can't afford it, you can't afford it, so why even cross your tourist Reeboks over the Valentino threshold? You're just going to be tempted and tortured and talked about. It is not within your budget; your money's no good there. So just stay away.

Living IRL (In Real Life, for Squares)

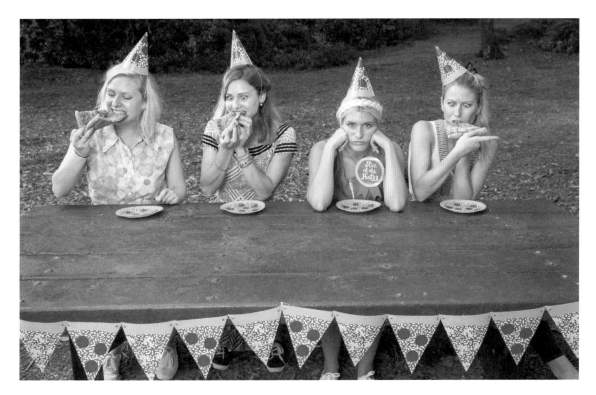

In *Calorie Accounting*, we're living our lives within the confines of a very specific—and oftentimes very tight—budget. We have successfully become en*light*ened *consumers* of the *market*place and know full well how to shop and cook for ourselves in a calorically conservative way, but what about when we have to leave the comforts of our own kitchens? Is it possible to stay on a diet *and* live life in the real world? I will be the first to admit that I'm really lousy at this, so for me, complete concentration on accounting for my calories means **cocooning**—cooping myself up and staying away from functioning society for whatever period of time the metamorphosis demands. (I realize that this is completely crazy and most people have way too much on their plates to commit to the doldrums of the monkish existence I find necessary for my own focus. I wouldn't recommend it. It's sociopathic. But I know myself, and how I tick, and I gotta do what I gotta do.) Anyway. Here's where I'm certainly no expert. But I know what I *should* be practicing if I wasn't a mental patient, so I'll preach it to you, and then at least one of us can get a life.

Restaurants. Going out to eat is more or less the number one reason to live. It's social, it's celebratory, it's satisfying. Dieting is so difficult because society places such a huge emphasis on food for human interactivity. When you're getting together with your girlfriends, you're going to go out to eat. You just are. What else is there to do? A movie? Well, you get dinner before or after, and if you don't, you sneak dinner into the theater in your purse. Shopping? Sbarro is going to flag you down for a break sooner or later. So what, are you gonna like, just go for a walk with someone through the forest preserves and talk about birds and pinecones? Get real. Who does that anymore? Whoever invited you to do that is a murderer.** If you're getting together with friends, you're going to put something in your mouth. So how can you stay accountable?

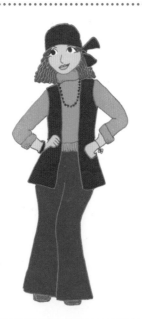

**   ** *Hippy Hippie Tip!*
If you are about to be murdered in a forest, pinecones in fact make excellent weapons. So scratchy. Go for the eyes!

- **Do your research.** Lots of times, we choose restaurants by grazing menus and making decisions based on price points. When you're Calorie Accounting, do the same thing, but assess the price in terms of what your caloric wallet can afford. If you know where you're going to eat ahead of time, look for the restaurant's menu online— you can decide what you're going to order, figure the caloric value, and budget your day accordingly.

- **Stick to the plan.** You've gone in knowing what you're going to order, so stay with it. Say no to the bread basket, skip the shared appetizer, and pretend everyone's got mono when they're all dipping their spoons into the communal mousse. You are strong and your friends are assholes for dangling these delights in your face, but just drink a lot of water so you have to excuse yourself to pee a lot and keep from bearing constant witness to their overeating evil.

- **Gross yourself out!** I saw Khloé Kardashian do this once on an episode of KUWTK. If you miscounted and thought you could afford that side of fries but really can't/shouldn't, then ruin it! Find something that you hate (for me, ketchup or mayo; your own spit will do, too) and smother those fries in that terrible condiment. Poof! Your craving is passed.

- **BYO/DIY.** Seriously, you may look like a loser now, but you're gonna look like hot shit soon, and then no one will judge you for the medicine cabinet of dietary supplements that travels in your purse. You want to save calories? Then bring your own and do it yourself! Order a salad with grilled chicken and vegetables and *that's it*, and then whip out your own measurement of your own favorite low calorie dressing, your own fat free feta or other lite cheese, and your own pre-counted pumpkin seeds to replace the crunch and saltiness of a crouton. Voila! You're out to eat without breaking the bank!

- **Hot breeds hot.** Order hot tea and sip in between courses. Hot liquid will keep your hunger under control, and as long as you have something to satisfy your oral fixation (find that old pacifier from your rave days!), you won't feel as tempted by the other things on the table. And obvs, no calories here.

Bars. Drinking is what made me so horribly, horribly fat. And it wasn't so much about the calories consumed whilst imbibing as it was about the massive amounts of food I would come home to when my brain wasn't capable of making healthy decisions. I'm talking stacks and stacks of microwaved quesadillas. Entire boxes of spaghetti doused in full sticks of butter and mountains of Parmesan cheese. Family-sized bags of peanut M&Ms. Mixing bowls of melted cheddar cheese, enjoyed with a spoon. And I wondered how on earth it all happened . . . anyway. For people with a little more will power than me, alcohol can be totally manageable on a diet. Here's how:

- **Drunk budgeting.** Calorie Accounting when drinking is a one-two punch. Not only do you obviously have to budget for the calories in each beverage consumed, but also for your alcohol tolerance. Each drink takes you closer and closer to the fuzzy line that, when crossed, prohibits you from making good choices. Know where that line is and you can stay safe on the other side. (This diet plan might be the answer to many a regretful morning in a stranger's bed!) If at three drinks you're slurring, it'll only take one more and you'll be slurping . . . cup after cup of Cup Noodle. So know exactly where you're going to cut yourself off and do it. Keep a tally on your hand! It's like the cool new henna tattoo.

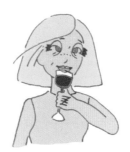

- **Bar rules.** Alcoholic drinks can be super caloric. Know your drink, know its calories, and know how many you're going to let yourself have before throwing back anything. In general, a glass of wine is around 100 calories, a beer is around 150, and a mixed drink with a no-calorie mixer (diet soda, soda water, NOT tonic), is around 65 calories. But be smart here. Yeah, you can have almost three Jack & Diets for the price of a Bud, but think about how drunk and stupid you'll be then. You can't afford *that* either.
- **Night cap.** If you're honest with yourself and know that when you come home after a night of drinking, no matter how tipsy you might or might not be, you're gonna want a snick-snack, then plan ahead. No harm in a little late-night nibble as long as it's not a stuffed crust pizza with a side of garlic knots. So before you go out, prepare your munchies. Put together a lovely platter of fruits and vegetables and have it sitting accessibly in the fridge, ready and waiting for when you come stumbling home. If you have to, you can even hide all the other food in the crisper. If you really have to, you can seal the crisper with packing tape. If you really, really have to, duct tape. Drunk's got nothing on duct, I promise.

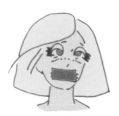

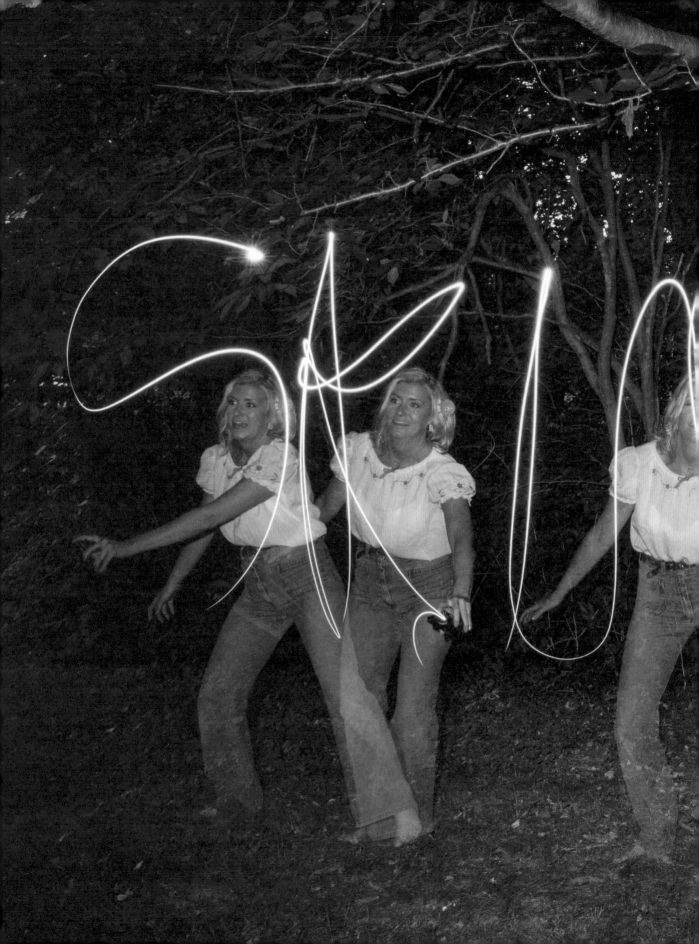

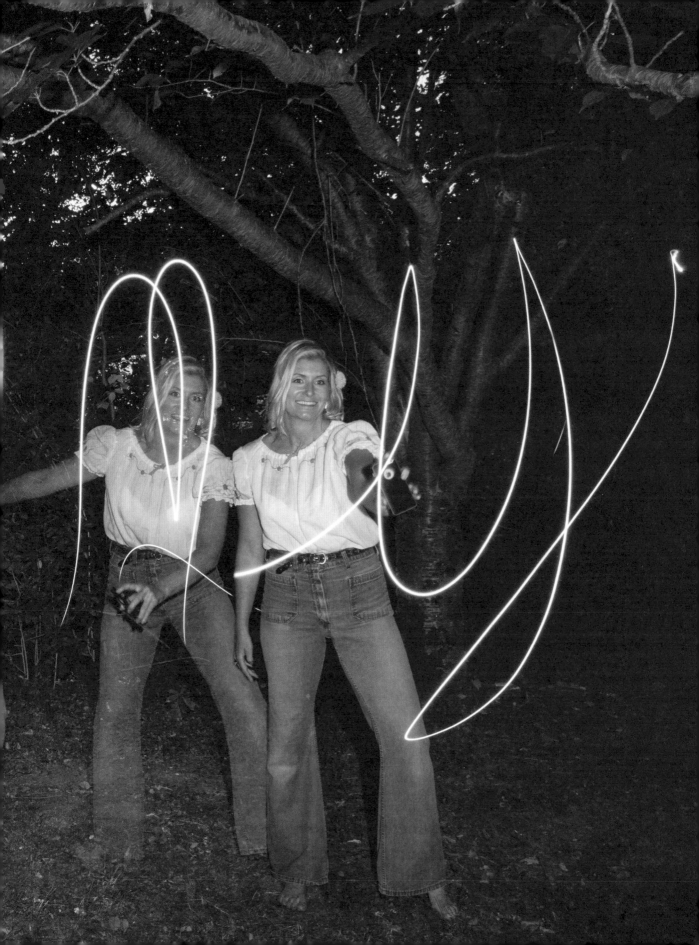

Suck It!

My step-great-aunt used to look me up and down disgustedly when I was an oft-plump teen starting to fall in love with all things vintage, especially the clothes. "They just didn't make your shape in those days," she would say. "You're a bigger gal, and you shovel your food. Trim ladies take their time."

Two things I wanted to say in response:

1. SUCK IT!
2. You should know; you haven't chewed on more than a cocktail onion in 23 years.

When my step-great-aunt saw me for the first time in a decade, after I had lost 33 pounds simply by Calorie Accounting, she nearly choked on her Manhattan: "I thought you would be so much heavier," she whimpered. "Also, I just love your vintage dress."

Well, the SUCK IT sentiment helped me more than she knew. Even if my angsty seventeen-year-old self didn't want to hear it, it was true that I shoveled—I was a pig. I ate like I was racing. I won three pie-eating contests, after all.

But as we've talked about before, "knowing yourself" is half the battle. I know I'm a serial snacker (and a cereal snacker, if we're talking about

Grape Nuts), and I know I tend to eat too fast. To combat the latter? I've learned to suck it! Suck your snack and you can enjoy it for longer. (I know, I know: That's what she said.) And stretching out the caloric intake for as long as you possibly can translates to tons of calories saved over time. Because time is money. And money is calories. And calories are all that we care about. You know how this works.

Things You Can Suck for a Long TIme:

- Hot Dogs
- Cocktail wieners
- Bratwurst
- Kielbasa
- Breakfast sausage

JK Haha ROFL No But for Real Though, Good Sucking Foods:

- Popsicles! Sugar free Popsicle brand: 15 calories; sugar free Creamsicle: 40 calories; low fat Fudgsicle: 60 calories; or make your own low calorie popsicles! Recipe on page TK.
- Hard candies! Werther's Original Sugar Free Caramel Hard Candies: 40 calories per five pieces (each piece lasts about five minutes—great movie snack!); Baskin Robbins Cookies 'n' Cream Hard Candy: 10 calories per piece
- Frozen berries/grapes: 80 calories per cup
- Hershey's Kisses: 22 calories per Kiss. BE CAREFUL! If you have willpower and you can stop when you mean to stop, you're fine

here. But if one morsel of true milk chocolate sends you scarfing, ignore this suggestion.

- David brand Dill Pickle flavored sunflower seeds: 160 calories per pack. There are other, less freakish, flavors, too.
- Ice, flavored with Crystal Light: 0–5 calories per tray. But only if you're alone; no one likes to hang out with an ice-chewer.

Not So Good Sucking Foods:

- Pineapple. Too much of this and your tongue will bleed from the acid.
- Salt & Vinegar Kettle Chips. Too much of this and you'll get the thrush.
- Fried cheese sticks. You'll choke and die.

See ya, suckers!!!!

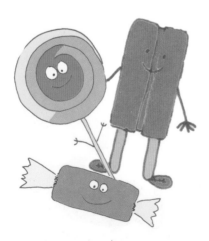

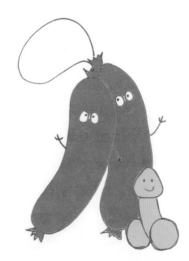

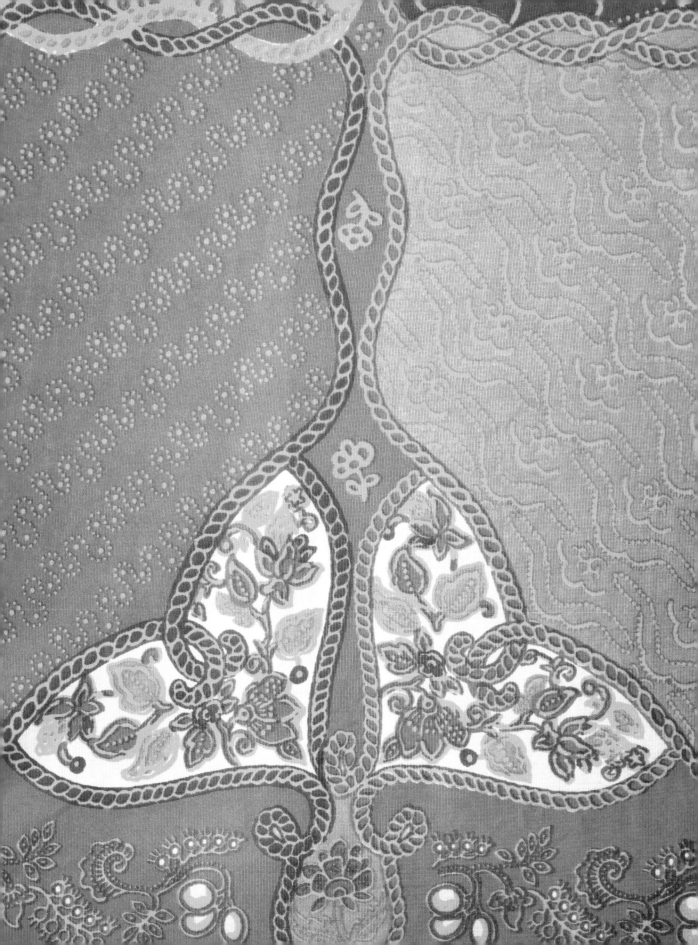

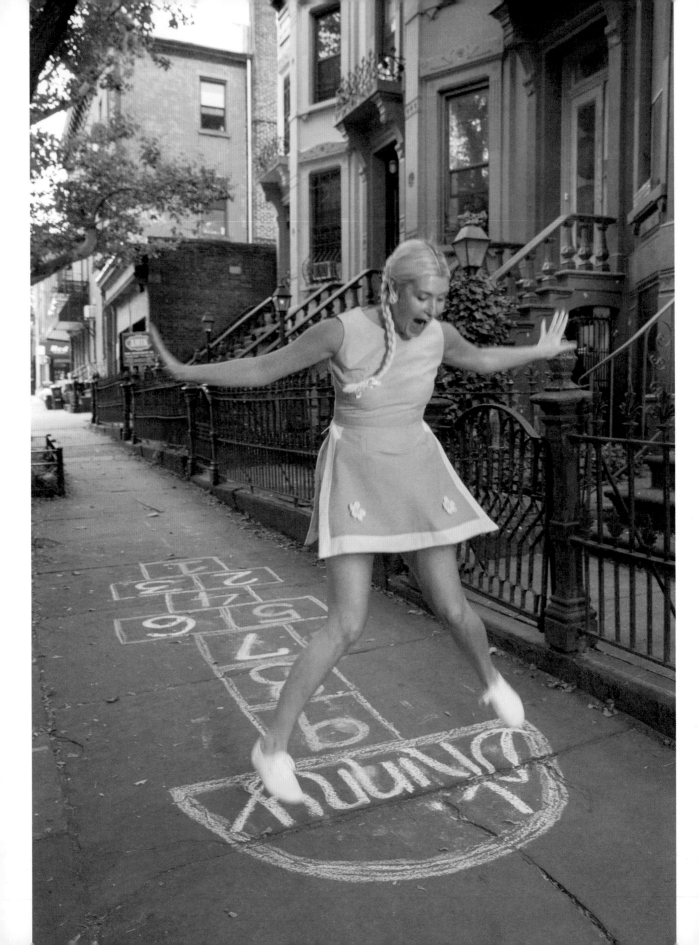

A Hop, Skip, and a Jump to Skinny

You already know from the 45 different kinds of diets you've tried that these things never exactly follow a straight line. It's always two steps forward, one step back, peaks and valleys, endless plateaus, roads to nowhere. Even in *Calorie Accounting*, you'll face these obstacles and the emotional rollercoasters that come with them. But because you're a seasoned loser, you know to keep the wind at your back and hop along. Trust the system, and you'll get to where you want to be.

Think of it like a game of hopscotch. You start with tiny goals: throw your rock, hop to it, check it off your list. Keep going: your goals get higher, harder. You need more balance and endurance to stay the course. You need precision to target and pursue your goals. You need to be swift on your feet, switching from hop to jump and back again. You return to START often, to remind yourself where you came from. You throw the rock again and again, every step placed so that you don't fall off. And then, before you know it, the game is over. You've won! You leap to your goal, dust off the chalk, and keep struttin' down that sidewalk like the skinny, sexy bitch you are.

Dear Dietry

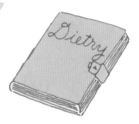

As you're taking progress photos with paper bags on your head, calculating all your daily checks and balances in your Loser Ledger, trying new recipes, new workouts, new Netflix binges, and altogether experiencing the awesome spectrum of human emotion in its entirety (such is dieting), it might be a good idea to take notes.

Keeping a "diet journal" is something a lot of *Today Show* nutritionists and Doctors Oz will regularly recommend, and for good reason: "Writing it down" keeps you grounded, organized, focused, and honest—it makes things official. Just as you disclosed to your 17-year-old diary that you finally got your period and could stop bringing red magic marker to school to feign feminine accidents, you can now disclose to your diet diary what you ate, how you feel, how your poop was, if you got any catcalls today, etc. As we all know, losing weight is hard. It's draining. And even if this particular program makes mathematical sense and is proven to work, that doesn't mean it's not a challenge to stay in the game. You can feel alone out there sometimes, and you wish you didn't have to do this stupid shit and that you could just have access to as much molly as Miley and you'd be naturally heroin chic forever, but it's not that way. We are real people, we have put on real weight, and we have to lose it in a real way. While you're on this journey, there'll be plenty of new ideas and breakthroughs and rage rants swimming up there in your head . . . so help yourself—be accountable to yourself—and get it all on paper.

Recently, I went back to my own Diet Diary from four years ago when I lost the weight. This first entry is from Day One: just another day on just another diet, depressed and defeated, going through the motions, hating everything:

Monday 2/8, 163 lbs

Today I ate . . .
egg beaters
2 links fake sausage
banana
sushi – cali rolls (prolly like 15 or something insane)
coffee
string cheese
100 cal popcorn
green tea

½ hour workout – treadmill/weights

I feel...
Disgusted with my weight
Hideous
Nervous about this thing on my arm
Desperate to get skinny in a healthy way

Good things about life:
— doing well at work
— found $10 bill in the bathroom today
— good friends

Tomorrow I will . . .
Work out
Work
Make valentines
Have a bunch of mini-meals:
— Egg Beaters/tomato/soy meat/grape nuts
— banana
— activia
— soup/salad
— sushi
— popcorn
Clean
Laundry

Good lord, is there anything more empty and depressing?? Looking back on my life at that point makes me sad :(But this second entry is the very next day—a complete turnaround. This is the honest-to-god moment that I discovered the joy of Calorie Accounting for the very first time, and knew that it would finally be cake* from here:

Tuesday 2/9

Today I ate . . .

— Egg Beaters—30cal
— soy bacon—60cal
— tomato—15cal

---

* Gluten-free zucchini cake.

- grape nuts—200cal
- coffee—5cal
- banana—110cal
- spicy shrimp spring roll—222cal
- spinach salad w/ ½ string cheese and 15 sprays balsamic salad spritzer—90cal
- chicken chili—250cal
- popcorn—100cal
- green tea—0
- spaghetti squash seeds (a bit of seasoned salt)—32cal

Okay. So say I burn 1500 calories/day just existing. Ballpark. Might be underestimating. Then all I should have to do is eat 1000 calories a day to make the difference 500/day, which is 3500/week, which I learned is a pound. Now. If I can burn 500 EXTRA calories a day with exercise, I should potentially be able to lose 2 pounds/week. Right?

1114 calories eaten – 1500 calories from existing – 169 cal from pilates = -555

I HAVE TO ALWAYS HAVE A DEFICIT OF AT LEAST 500 CALORIES/DAY

And then this is simple!

I WOULD LIKE TO TRY TO HAVE A DEFICIT OF 1000 CALORIES/DAY

But. You haven't messed up as long as you're 500 in the hole per day. NBD.

Today I feel . . .
Happy about the math in the diet
Like I had a VERY productive day—snow day, didn't leave the house. Did work, cleaned, valentines and misc. correspondence, laundry, made spaghetti squash . . . all sorts of things.
Feel good about what I can eat if it's really the case.
Feel good about not having to be . . . unhealthy.
Had a nice conversation w/ dad
Feel really good about not sending Mike a desperate Valentine as I was planning . . . Feel excited about concentrating on me.
Pilates wasn't so hard today. Almost didn't work out. Remember that it's not so bad.

Tomorrow . . .
Same food all day . . . maybe measure your grape nuts . . .
It'll be helpful not to have that sushi
Remember portion control . . . be proud of your dinner portions tonight.
Go to the gym in the morning
Close a deal
Go to fancy Kroger IF you close a deal
Classic Rock mixtape

MAKE IT RAIN, LEVY!!!!

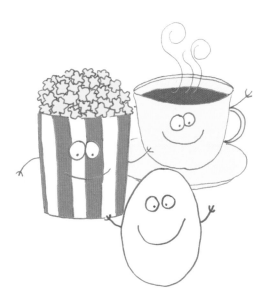

I remember going back to entry #2 again and again, whenever things got tough. It was such a huge help to have that breakthrough written down, on the record, in real time. And I continued to write my daily entries, checking in with myself, telling the truth to myself. Maybe I was scared for weigh-in tomorrow. So I'd write about why (was it the entire stuffed crust pizza I ate last night?), and what I was going to do next week to feel better. Maybe I was stoked that I ran four miles straight while watching *Kourtney and Kim Take Miami*, and knew I wanted a pat on the back, but had to put ink on paper to promise to myself that I wouldn't eat a whole Key lime pie in celebration. Maybe I just wanted to get it down in writing, in big red bold letters, that I lost 8.5 pounds in my first three weeks of Calorie Accounting! And maybe I had an idea for a book, and didn't want to lose it . . . :)

Let your brain dictate the same thoughts and put it on the record. Include a food log, a workout tracker, a weight loss graph, shopping lists, things to do, notes to self, ideas you found in *Self* magazine, ideas you found in *US Weekly*, inventions, names for pets, lists of go-to karaoke songs, dreams, movies to see, vacations to take. . . . Your mind is running wild and your life is filled to the brim, so keep up and stay tuned in. Jot it down and you'll never forget to remember how far you've come.

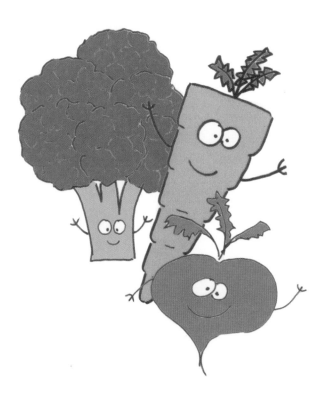

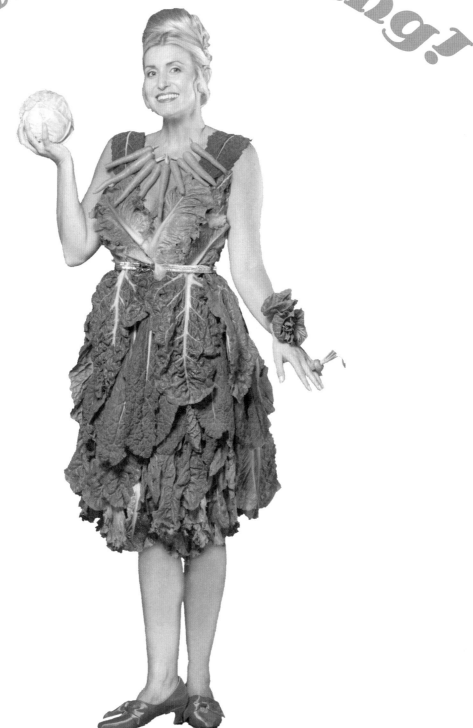

Salad Dressing!

Pretend it's high school again and your parents have just given you $200 to run off to the mall and put your dream prom ensemble together. SO EXCITING!!! You haven't had this kind of loot in your hands since you stole it out of your mom's purse last week! So many possibilities, so many details, so much to consider! You need to look like a princess, a movie star, an angel sent from heaven . . . and most importantly you need to look like someone who's ready to give it up pronto to Bryan O'Gregory. Where to begin??

Here's how it all works itself out after mall madness:

Dress: $70
Shoes: $30
Corsage: $10
Necklace: $15
Earrings: $10
Clutch: $15
Custom vajazzle: $20
Tiara: $25

You even have an extra $5 for a slice at Sbarro or a condom! Oh gee, prom's going to be magical!!!

Flash forward 15 years: Prom happened, and maybe so did the conception of Bryan Jr., and the baby weight and the Sbarro have been hanging on to your magical love handles ever since. No worries, that's why you're here with me! Let's take what we learned about dressing on a budget way back when, and now we'll apply it to dressing . . . salad!

350 calories would make for a nice light lunch . . . let's see what we can do.

Spinach (3 cups): 21 calories
Grape tomatoes (10): 20 calories
Lite string cheese (pulled/shredded, 1 stick): 50 calories
Avocado (1/4 fruit): 70 calories
Cucumber (1 cup slices): 16 calories
Broccoli (1/2 cup): 15 calories
Chickpeas (1/2 cup): 110 calories
Paul Newman Lite Balsamic Vinaigrette (2 tbsp): 45 calories
Salt-N-Pepa: 0 calories

Boom! 347 delicious calories! The most beautiful salad in the world, skimpin' on nothin'! You get to have your cheese, you get to have your avocado, you get to have your chickpeas . . . and it all fits perfectly into your budget. Did you run an extra mile on the treadmill today? Throw a Reese's Peanut Butter Cup on top for a well-earned 105 extra calories. Or 50 extra grape tomatoes. Or another quarter avocado. Or two more packages of string cheese. Or do NOTHING, and pocket an extra 100 calories for a rainy day!

Cha-ching! Cha-chomp.

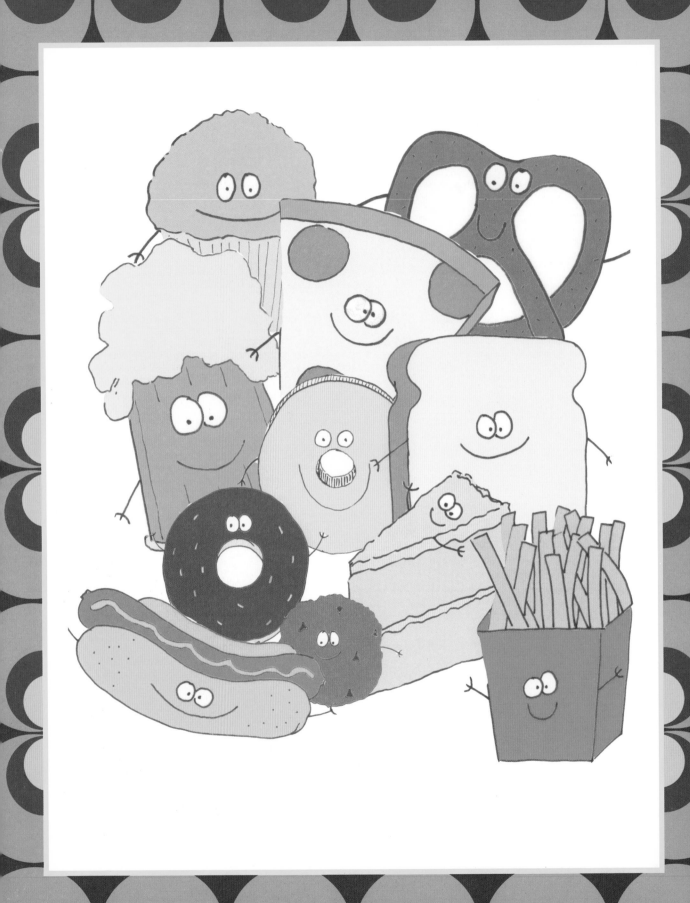

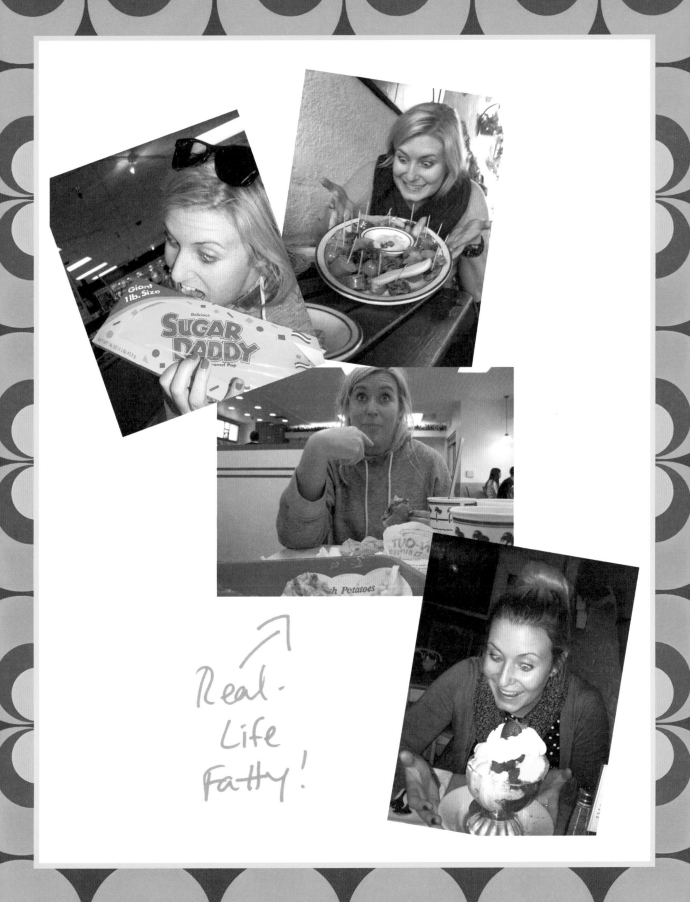

Real.
Life
Fatty!

Embezzlement

As Billy Joel so astutely sang, crashing his Audi into a corner bodega for the third or fourth time, *You're only human / it's okay to fuck up.* Or something to that effect. And it's true, Billy. We *are* only human. And since we, who are reading this book, happen to be a bunch of fatty humans, we know exactly where our downfalls are going to come into play. We're gonna break. We're gonna binge. We're gonna wanna kill ourselves about it. But chin up, round spectacle. Remember that second wind.

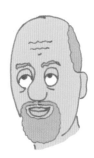

In Calorie Accounting, we consider **embezzlement** a punishable crime. It's messing up and stealing from your own savings account to try to make up the difference, thereby submerging yourself into even hotter water and deeper debts. Happens to the best of us. You've been working hard to build up a sustainable and reputable business—this business of dieting—and you're saving and spending just as you should be, maintaining your budget, working towards goals, being smart and conservative, being successful . . . but you're starting to get a little impatient. You're losing a pound here, a pound there, but when will your fortune come in? When will you finally be the picture of perfection that your driver's license weight suggests? And then, suddenly, your desperate daydream is interrupted when a perfect slice of New York style strawberry cheesecake presents itself to your hungry eyes, plate and fork and all. And you think to yourself, *I had a nice long run on the treadmill today. . . I can probably afford a bite or two.* And you take a bite or two. And a third for good luck. And then. You want more. So what do you do? You do what we all do. We panic in the face of adversity, of temptation. We are humans and we buckle under the pressure. (Another Billy Joel classic!) We lie. We cheat. We steal. We eat that cheesecake and we order another one. À la mode. And then we come home and we eat everything in the fridge, because hey, we've blown it anyway, so why not just go to town and get in on every little calorie we've been missing all this time!? Sound familiar? Such a splurge is criminal, yes, but maybe only a misdemeanor if you can keep your maniacal behavior down to a freak outburst and away from a full-blown spending spree. As long as you can commit yourself to change and do your time for the crime, you can erase this little mishap from your record. Bernie Madoff should be so lucky.

Debt Solutions

Whether you charged a pair of Louboutins to your emergency credit card, you're paying off student loans from clown school, or you bought a house ever, you know what it means to be in the red. You've got bills that you can't afford to pay. And likewise, maybe last night was 25¢ wings night at the bar next door and you forgot which currency you were supposed to be frugal with. You ate 3,000 calories worth of buffalo chicken

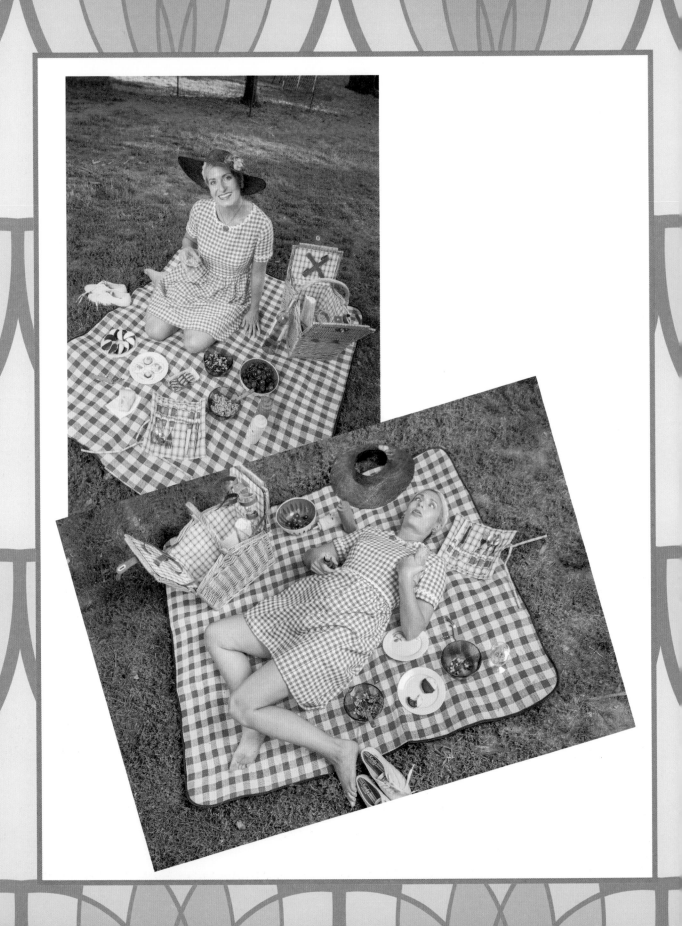

and blue cheese, but according to your Loser Ledger, this was nowhere *near* what you had budgeted for. Well, this sucks, but this happens. And IT'S OKAY. Do you hear me? You must hear me. I need you to hear me. IT'S OKAY!!! You can screw up every once in a while, and you don't have to stick your finger down your throat to repent. (And seriously, don't even try with buffalo chicken. Your nose will probably bleed.) Just drink a bunch of water, take a deep breath, know that you enjoyed your wings, and go to bed. Tomorrow is a new day. And when you wake up . . .

If you're like me (and I think this could potentially be a freakish mutation, but perhaps I'm not alone), one "off-meal" (or off-*day* if I'm really being honest, because as much as I may preach, if I screw up once I'll be on a free-for-all till the stroke of midnight) will almost always translate to an immediate 5–7 pound weight gain the next morning. It is completely insane. It makes me lose my mind. Granted, this is not real weight—this is bloat and water and junk I haven't pooped out yet—but it's enough to send me reeling in regret. And I have three choices: 1) I could order a pizza and say to hell with this diet; 2) I could change course and put myself on any number of get-thin-quick schemes, like a liquid cleanse, Slim-Fast, or anorexia (this all guarantees immediate misery and subsequent cellulite); or 3) I could get right back on the Calorie Accounting horse and **GET TO THE GYM AS SOON AS POSSIBLE.**

The gym, or "The Bank," or whatever (I'm getting lost in my own metaphors . . . and here comes another one!), is like the morning-after pill of unprotected bingeing. Kill that calzone baby in your stomach as soon as you are able with double-time on the treadmill. You may not be able to b*earn* back every single calorie in just one session, but you can make a definite difference and get yourself back on the abstinence track. For

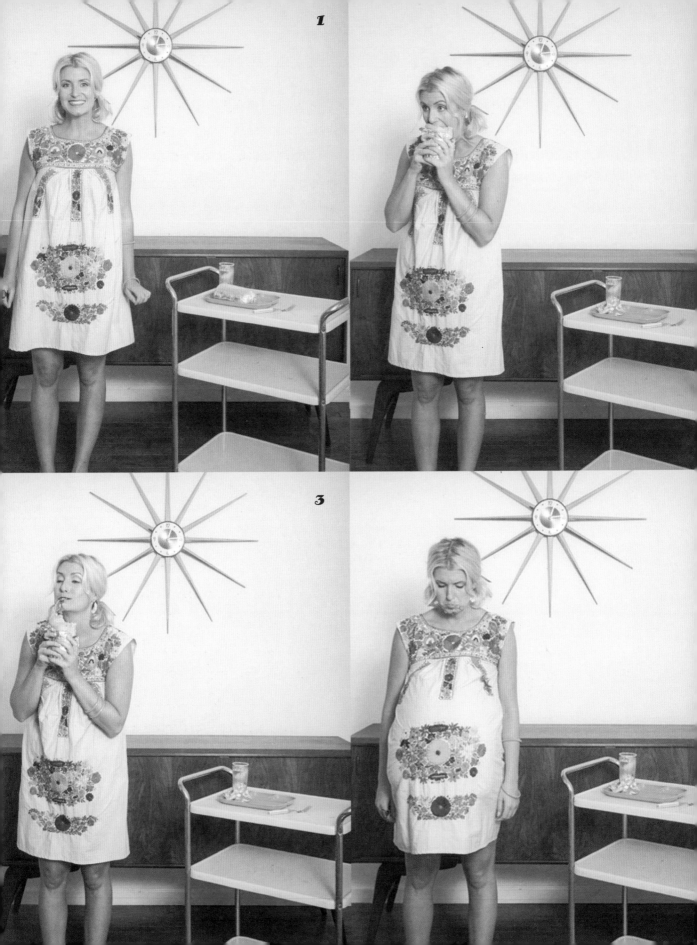

every day of eating out of your budget, you can expect two days of pay-back to get back in the black. So if you binge on a Friday and a Saturday, it will take four days of your regular diet to get back to where you were pre-breakdown. A week at an all-inclusive resort in Jamaica will take two weeks of steadfast scrimping to be back to normal, ready to take on new goals and benchmarks. Just so long as you realize the severity and length of your sentence and respect the law, there's no reason why you can't order the cheese sticks every once in a while.

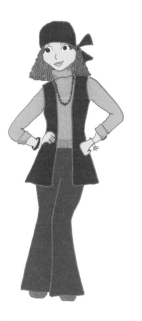

** *Hippy Hippie Tip!*

Speedy delivery! While a good workout and a swift return to your regimen is the only real way to get back in the black, it might help you stay focused if you could lighten up a bit. Swiss Kriss Herbal Laxatives and prune juice are two very organic, very healthy options for gettin' a move on, if you know what I mean.

For a Song

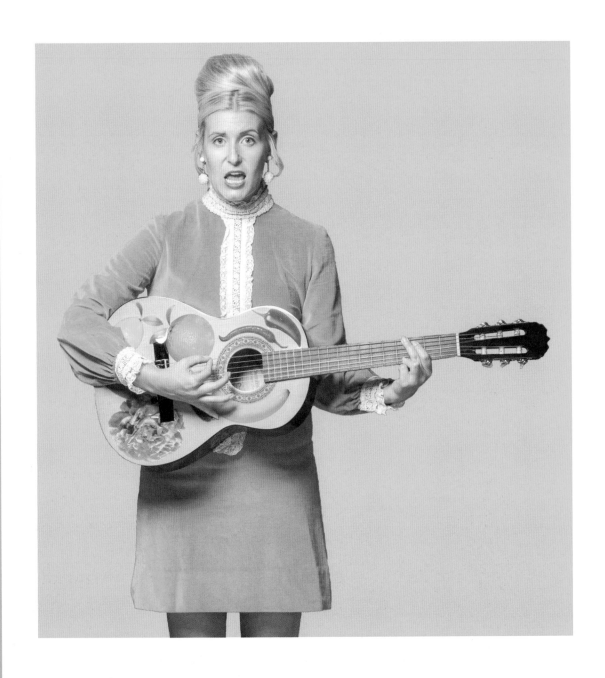

(To the tune of Britney Spears's "Oops!...I Did It Again")

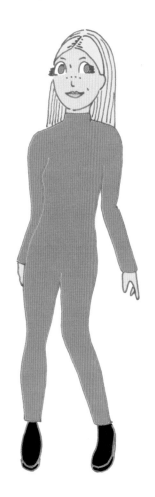

I think I ate it again—
I microwaved up
Some hot slop and cheese.
Oh fatty,
It might taste like a dream,
But it's not worth the cals
When you can't zip your jeans.
Oh to lose all this jiggle,
And unleash a skinnier me!
Oh fatty, fatty,
Oops! I ate it again
I shoveled some snacks, got lost in TV,
Oh fatty fatty,
Oops! I've fucked it all up,
Might as well stuff my face…
I'll start – to – morrow.

*Fun fact:

When I was in my golden teenage diet years in high school (I gained 20 pounds when I turned 16 and started eating bagels every day for breakfast *and* lunch, tried to lose it by eating exclusively grapes for two weeks, passed out D. J. Tanner-style at badminton practice, eventually found success with Atkins), I used to fawn over the Britney Spears "Oops!" music video on TRL, and a real-life incentive for me was the possibility of owning her red vinyl cat suit and using it as a "goal" outfit—if I could fit into that, I thought, I would be officially fit. However, after a half-eaten piece of Justin Timberlake's French toast sold at auction for $100,000, I was discouraged.

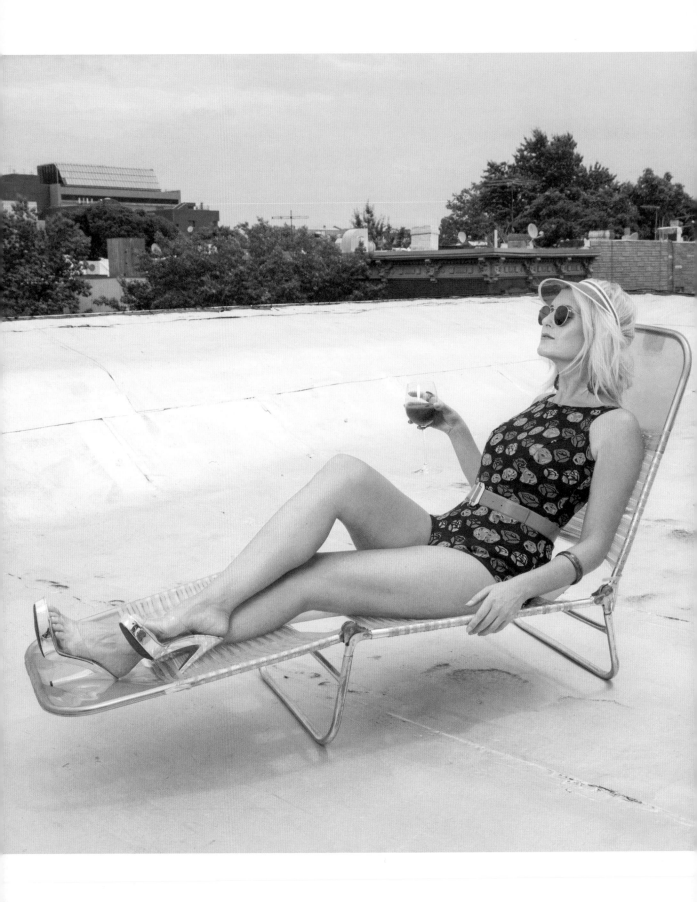

When All's Accounted For

Losing weight is a completely insane experience. Textbook bipolar. Manic depressive. The up days are so awesome you want to scream from the tops of mountains about how your skinny jeans zip again, and the down days are so awful you want to casino-buffet yourself to certain death. But hopefully by now you've learned that the best part of Calorie Accounting is the *knowing*: The absolute assuredness that in the end, when all our numbers have been crunched, this will work. Faith in math. Easy as pie. Mmmmm . . .

Hungry? This brings me to our next point.

Success. Sweet, sweet success. A loooong time coming and so well-deserved, real and tangible success can either be the gateway to a whole new life of health and fitness and happiness, or could, conversely, be the worst thing to happen to a dieter who's not ready for it. The latter is what one might call **The Hammertime Effect.** Like the Reverend MC himself, you've taken your beat-up-broke-down ass from rags to riches, catapulting into fame and fortune faster than you can say *U Can't Touch This.* You've had a single goal in mind for weeks, months, maybe even years. You've scrimped and saved and sacrificed and deprived yourself, and now that you finally have this "thing," this holy grail of hotness that you've been reaching for all this time, you haven't the slightest idea what to do with it. Hammer went mental. He realized he made a gazillion

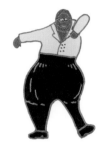

dollars and completely freaked out. Panicked. Snapped. He'd never had this kind of dough before, and clearly his financial advisors were distracted by his golden balloon pants, because his instantaneous reaction was to buy up everything he could get his hands on. Mansions, yachts, private jets, diamond grills, more bubble pants, livestock, mass quantities of Ovaltine, you name it. And what happened? He went bankrupt. One day of being rich doesn't mean you've won The Economy Game, and one day of being thin doesn't mean you've won The Diet Game. It's not a game. There is no end. It's a lifestyle, a stock market, ever-changing, and you're invested. Of course success deserves celebration. And you're so fresh out of the drive-thru that a little fatty residue might still be lingering in your newly thin frame . . . and the porker within equates celebration with what? That's right. Food. And lots of it. But look at your Loser Ledger. Observe the numbers. Understand the math. Look at your weekly naked pixx with the stickers on your head! Look at that first one and try to hold back the vomit rising in your throat. Was that even you? It's incredible how hard you've worked and how far you've come. Is it really worth it to freak out and Hammertime your way back into bloating? One irresponsible calorie splurge can lead to another, and another, and a few days of celebration turns into a few weeks, and then suddenly your party dress is bruising your ribcage and you're not feeling so celebratory anymore. Before you know it, you'll go bankrupt, and then you'll either have to start the whole damn thing over again, or you'll have to become a portly preacher. The choice is yours.

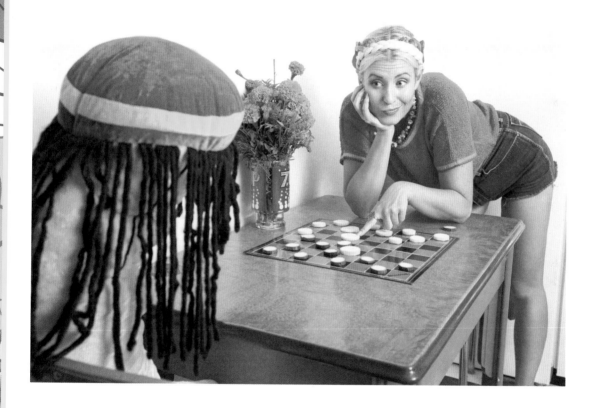

So how, then, will you manage to maintain the wealth of health for years to come? Simple. Just stay on budget. Our coveted Calorie Accounting equation works to calculate all forms of weight control—losing, gaining, and maintaining. Once you've arrived at your goal weight, all you have to do each day is net your BMR and you'll stay put on that scale. (For all you theater majors, this means matching your BMR to break even after tabulating what you eat and what you burn.) And remember! Your BMR changes as your weight does, so check it again once you've reached your goal.

You can have a cheat meal here and there, treat yourself just a little more often, but be sure to remember our little lesson on embezzlement—own up to your mistakes and do your time for any crime. One day of being bad = two days of being good, and then you're right back on track. It's no big deal if you look at it that way, and if you continue to live by the proven math, you're golden. It's a fact. So be cool. Know your numbers. Respect them. Believe them. Remember your journey. Remember what it felt like when you couldn't fit into anything in your closet, or when you counted four chins in a rapidly un-tagged Facebook photo. Remember what it felt like the day your cutoffs looked like cutoffs again, and not some kind of denim sausage casing. Or when your friends first said, "You look great." Be proud of who you've become, and be wary of who you were letting yourself turn into. Be accountable. Be Calorie Accountable. Be awesome. Be you.

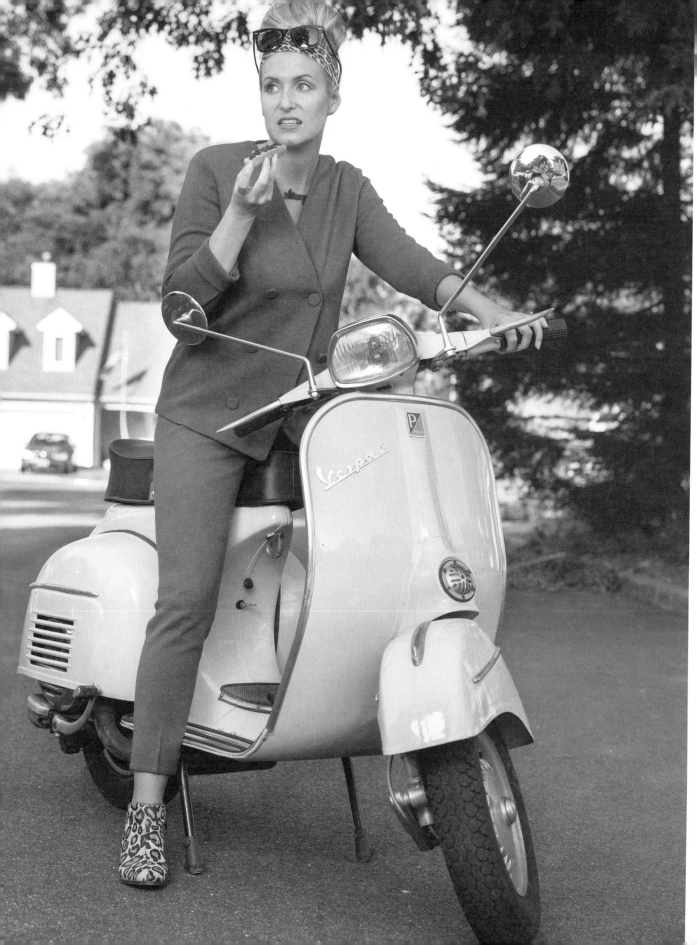

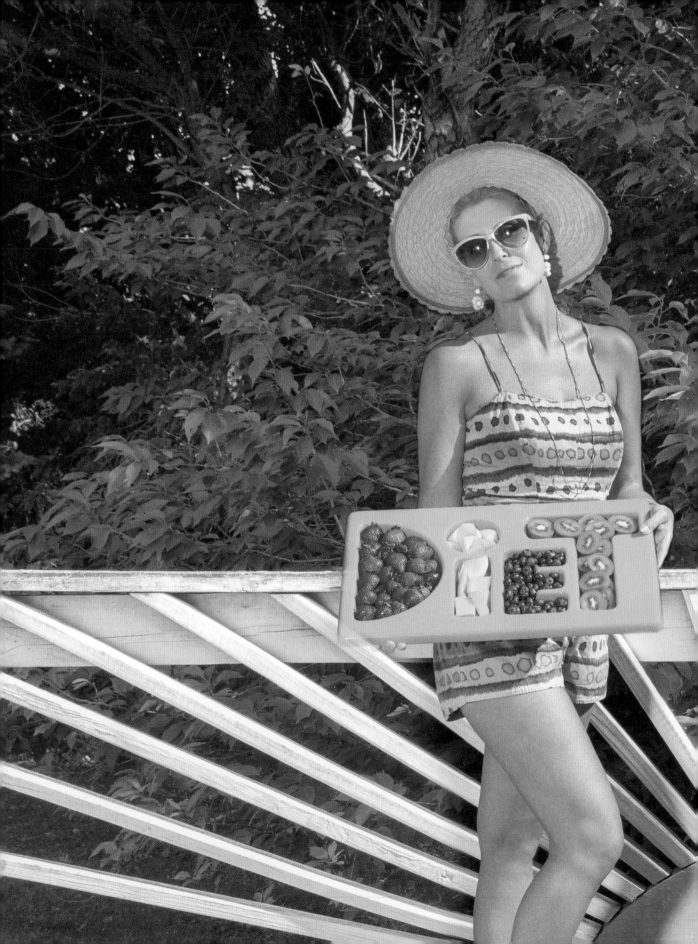

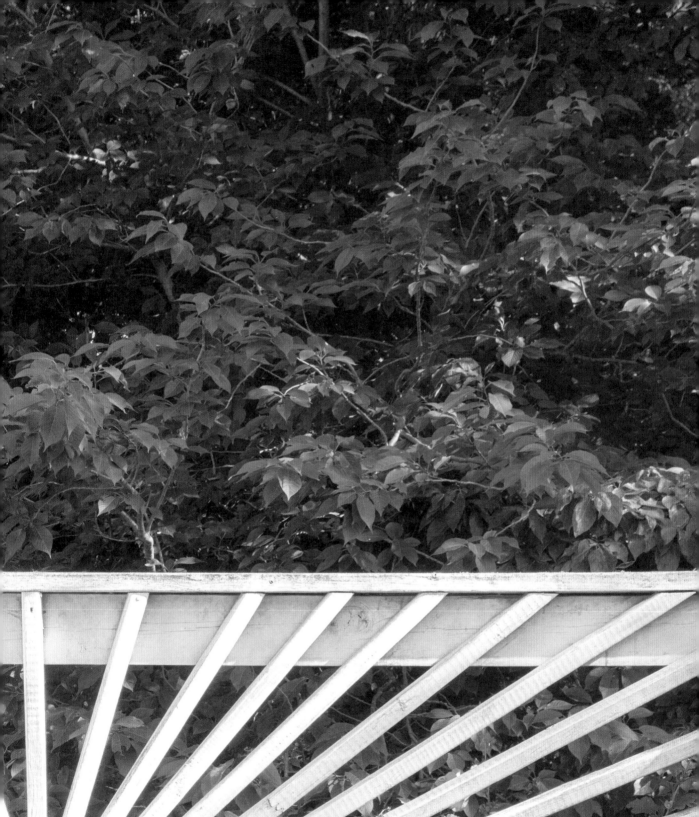

Recipes!

Here's a sampling of embarrassingly simple food concoctions I have created and shoved down my maw to much pleasure. Some are snacks, some are meals, some are desserts, some are drinks. Most everything's set up for a single serving, but a handful of options allow for sharing and/or a social life—if not, just a few nights' worth of lonely grazing. The calorie counts range from 30 to 360, and you can feel free to adjust however you wish: I've included calorie counts for each element of each recipe, so you can go more or less with whichever ingredient however you like. Salt to taste, calories to budget.

1. "Taffy Apple" — 140 calories

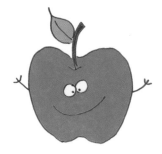

Prep: 1.5 minutes
Total time: 1.5 minutes
Yield: 1 snick-snack

Ingredients
1 Sugar Free Caramel Snack Pack (60 calories)
1 Granny Smith apple (80 calories)

Directions
Take Sugar-Free Caramel Snack Pack out of fridge. Open it. Take one washed Granny Smith apple and cut into eighths (or fourths, depending

on how big your mouth is and how bad you wanna house this thing). Arrange apple slices on cute plate with opened Snack Pack in the middle. Take out to living room and turn on *Jeopardy!* Dip slices into pudding and relax with Alex. (If you're feeling salty, you can sprinkle a little sea salt on your pudding, too, because salted caramel is #trending right now.)

2. Blueberry Soup — 83 calories

Prep: 30 seconds
Cook: 1.5 minutes
Total time: 2 minutes
Yield: 1 dessert/snick-snack

Ingredients
1 cup fresh blueberries (83 calories)
1 packet Stevia (0 calories)

Directions
Dump a washed bushel of fresh blueberries into a microwave-safe bowl. Take a fork or a spoon and lightly mash blueberries, until about half of them are popped. Stick bowl in microwave (you might cover with a paper towel if you don't want purple explosions all over your micro-wave), zap on high for 90 seconds. During this time you can take a quick wee or pluck a stray eyebrow. When timer goes off, remove bowl from microwave—*Achtung*! Could be HOT!—and mash hot blueber-ries a little more, to a liquidy pulp. Leave a few whole berries for the illusion of a pie-filling-like confection. Open pack of Stevia, sprinkle atop your soup, stir, and go to town! If you can afford it, add a dollop of fat free Cool Whip for a 15-calorie à la mode bonus. (To earn it, you

can run in place for 1.5 minutes while your soup is microwaving instead of tending to your brows.)*

3. Jicks 'n' Guac — 109 calories per serving (8 servings total)

Prep: 20 minutes
Inactive: 30–40 minutes
Total time – 1 hour
Yield: snacks for all 8 nights of Hanukkah

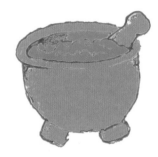

Ingredients
4 ripe avocados (560 calories)
1 bunch green onions, chopped (30 calories)
1 4 oz can Ortega Diced Green Chiles (20 calories)
Juice of 1 lime (0 calories)
Cilantro, if you can handle it (I have that disease where it tastes like soap) (10 calories)
Lawry's Seasoned Salt (0 calories)
White pepper (0 calories)
1 jicama, sliced (253 calories)

Directions
For the guac:
Slice, peel, and pit four avocados, throw meat in mixing bowl. Wash and chop green onions; add to bowl. Dump can of green chilies in, too. Chop and sprinkle cilantro if you like it okay. Squeeze half a lime and

---

* Those babies BLUE right through you! Remember to stay near a toilet when you're eating mass quantities of blueberries . . . nature's colonic!

sprinkle seasoned salt and white pepper to taste. Mash and mix and sample, adding lime juice and salt if it still needs a lil' something. Feel free to throw jalapenos or hot sauce or tomatoes in, too, if you want; this is just the way I do it, okay? Okay.

For the chips:
Jicama! (I have no idea where to find this in the grocery store, or how to identify it in its natural, raw form. I just know I've ordered this at Mexican restaurants instead of chips, and they've obliged.) Peel (I'm guessing?) and slice half the bulb into "chips." Dip them chips into that guac and taste all your dreams come true! To lighten things up even more—or, if you freak out at the grocery store and give up looking for jicama, as I have done many times myself—turn to cucumber instead. Each medium cuke is just 47 cals. Get at it!

4. Crunchy Munchie — 200 Calories

Prep: 1.5 minutes
Total time: 1.5 minutes
Yield: 1 light lunch/snick-snack

Ingredients
1 brown rice cake (60 calories)
1/2 medium avocado (140 calories)
Salt-N-Pepa to taste (0 calories)

Directions
This one's great if you need a crunchy, creamy, salty fix when you're high on the ganja. Untwist twist tie from rice cake bag. Remove one cake.

Place on cute dish. Cut ripe medium avocado in half. Remove skin and pit with paring knife; do not remove your finger. Spread half the avocado onto rice cake (you can save the other half in a plastic baggie with the pit to delay browning). Sprinkle kosher salt and black pepper on top to taste. For mad munchies, use two cakes, the whole avocado, and double the calories. Add tomato slices for an extra six calories if you're feeling wild.

5. Bare Waldorf — 184 Calories

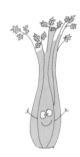

Prep: 4 minutes
Total time: 4 minutes
Yield: 1 snicky-snack

Ingredients
4 celery stalks (24 calories)
2 wedges Laughing Cow Creamy White Swiss (70 calories, 35 each)
¼ cup red grapes, halved (26 calories)
¼ cup Gala apples, chopped (16 calories)
1 tbsp chopped walnuts (48 calories)

Directions
Wash and dry celery. Cut into 6-inch logs. You can work with as many stalks of celery as you want; these calories are almost non-existent (6 per stalk!). Spread cheese wedges into celery canals (gross). Arrange halved grapes and chopped apples atop the cheese spread. Sprinkle walnuts. Admire attractive snicky-snack. Think about how you're gonna get skinnier than Serena; SCARF SHAMELESSLY!
xoxo, Diet Girl

6. Hot Slop — 282 Calories

Prep: 5 minutes
Cook: 10 minutes
Total time: 15 minutes
Yield: 1 trough of hot slop for 1 lil' piggy

Ingredients
½ cup firm tofu (88 calories)
1 10 oz bag frozen spinach (88 calories)
½ cup Ragu No-Sugar-Added Tomato & Basil Pasta Sauce (60 calories)
¼ cup Kraft Fat-Free Mozzarella (46 calories)
Hot sauce (0 calories)
I Can't Believe It's Not Butter spray (0 calories)

Directions
Dump entire bag of frozen spinach into saucepan and steam till thawed. Cut ¼ of the block of tofu out of the tofu box. Chop into small ½-inch cubes. Meanwhile, heat up a few tablespoons of I Can't Believe It's Not Butter spray in a saucepan, add tofu, and sauté. As tofu turns golden brown, dump thawed spinach and 1 cup of marinara on top. Let sizzle for 3–4 minutes, stirring. When everything's hot, dump into a bowl and sprinkle fat-free mozzarella on top. Douse in hot sauce and a dash of grated Parmesan cheese. Mix everything up to create an unidentifiable Christmas-colored slop. Change quickly into comfy-cozies, turn on *Keeping up with the Kardashians,* and enjoy!

7. Wing Night (Not!) — 64 Calories

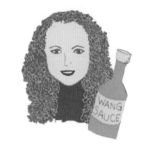

Prep: 2 minutes
Total time: 2 minutes
Yield: enough dinner to last through one episode
of *Felicity*

Ingredients
1 cup grape tomatoes (30 calories)
1 large cucumber, peeled (34 calories; if you're too lazy to peel and leave
skin on, it's 46 calories)
Frank's RedHot Buffalo Sauce (0 calories)

Directions
Wash a bushel of grape tomatoes. Throw in a bowl. Peel 1–2 cucumbers and slice into 1/2-inch thick medallions. Throw in the same bowl. Pour as much freaking zero-calorie buffalo sauce as you want into a lil' dipping dish. Take out to living room. Find an episode of *Felicity* on Netflix, dip your crudités in your hot sauce, and imagine you're eating 25¢ buffalo wings at the sports bar down the street as you work through internal conflicts about Noel versus Ben.

8. Watermelon Faux-jito — 51 Calories (per glass)

Prep: 2 minutes
Total time; 2 minutes
Yield: 2 drinks

Ingredients

2 cups watermelon, pureed (90 calories)
1 can Fresca (0 calories)
¼ cup fresh mint (12 calories)
Ice (0 calories)

Directions

Take 2 cups cubed watermelon and throw into a blender. Puree until smooth. Fill 2 tall, summery glasses (probably from Anthropologie) with ice. Distribute watermelon juice equally into glasses. Top off with *delicious Fresca zero-calorie citrus soda*! Garnish with a fresh mint leaf. If you have straws—preferably the hard plastic kind shaped like hearts or stars, or even leftover penis ones from a bachelorette party—it really completes the "fancy drink" feeling.

9. Thin-N-Out Animal Style Burger — 288 Calories

Prep: 5 minutes
Cook: 3 minutes
Total time: 8 minutes
Yield: 1 din-din

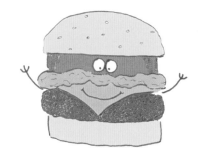

Ingredients

1 100-calorie hamburger bun (100 calories)
1 Original Gardenburger patty (110 calories)
1 slice Kraft Singles Fat Free Cheddar (25 calories)
1 tbsp Kraft Fat Free Thousand Island Dressing (25 calories)
I Can't Believe It's Not Butter spray (0 calories)
5 Claussen Dill Pickle Chips (5 calories)

1 slice tomato (5 calories)
¼ cup chopped white onion (17 calories)
1 leaf Bibb lettuce (1 calorie)

Directions

Jessica Alba says she ate an In-N-Out Burger right before the Golden Globes? Here's what she really had. Heat up some I Can't Believe It's Not Butter spray on a skillet and add chopped white onions. Sauté. Spread fat free Thousand Island dressing on both halves of a 100-calorie bun. Take a fake frozen burger from the breakfast aisle (I like Gardenburger the best), microwave it, throw it on the bun. Add a slice of fat free cheddar cheese to the hot patty and let it melt. Then top with lettuce, tomato, sautéed onion, and pickle chips. Squirt a little more dressing on top if you can afford it and dig in! Just as delicious (and nowhere near as dangerous) as that West Coast classic. Wanna save 100 calories? Do it up "protein style" and forget the bun—just wrap in lettuce. Look out, Alba!

10. Peppermint Hot Chocolate — 61 Calories

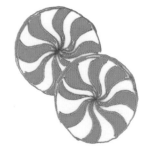

Prep: 30 seconds
Cook: 2 minutes
Total time: 2.5 minutes
Yield: 1 dessert

Ingredients
1 pouch Diet Swiss Miss Hot Chocolate (26 calories)
2 Brach's Sugar Free Starlight Mints (20 calories)
2 tbsp Fat Free Cool Whip (15 calories)

Directions

Dump out packet of Diet Swiss Miss in adorable wintry mug. Mix powder with water and microwave for however long it tells you to microwave it for. Unwrap two starlight mints. Plip-plop them into hot chocolate when it's done microwaving. Stir until mints dissolve. Top off with dollop of Cool Whip and enjoy this sinful nightcap while you cyberstalk your ex's new pudgy girlfriend.

11. Chik-skinn-A — 290 Calories

Prep: 1.5 minutes
Cook: 2.5 minutes
Total Time: 4 minutes
Yield: 1 din-din sandie

Ingredients
1 100-calorie bun (100 calories)
1 Morningstar Farms breaded chicken patty (140 calories)
5 Claussen Dill Pickle Chips (5 calories)
2 tbsp fat free honey mustard dressing (35 calories)
½ tsp Kraft Original BBQ Sauce (10 calories)

Directions

Take fake frozen chicken patty out of box and microwave it for however long. While it's zapping, mix honey mustard and BBQ sauce in a little bowl. Spread mixture onto each side of a 100-calorie sandwich bun. When chicken's ready, plop onto dressed bun and decorate with pickle chips. Put the top back on, smash it all down, and enjoy!

12. Buffauxlo Chicken Salad — 326 Calories

Prep: 1.5 minutes
Cook: 2.5 minutes
Total Time: 4 minutes
Yield: enough salad for half an episode of any original Netflix series

Ingredients
3 cups arugula (18 calories)
5 Morningstar Buffalo Wings (200 calories)
2 tbsp Wish-Bone Fat Free Blue Cheese Dressing (30 calories)
¼ cup Kraft Fat Free Shredded Cheddar Cheese (45 calories)
½ cup grape tomatoes, halved (15 calories)
¼ cup celery, chopped (5 calories)
¼ cup carrots, chopped or julienned (13 calories)

Directions
If you can afford the extra calories, you can shove this all into a 100-calorie tortilla and make yourself a freaking delicious buffalo chicken wrap, but to save yourself an extra mile at the gym, do it in salad form. Buy a thing of arugula from the store. Dump it in a bowl. Microwave five of the little Morningstar buffalo chicken nugget guys. Meanwhile, rinse and chop your veggies. When the chiXen is ready, cut it into halves or quarters. Be careful! Fake meat gets weirdly hot. Like, hotter than anything that occurs in nature. You can either refrigerate the fake meat and wait 30 to 60 minutes to throw it in the salad and chow down, or, if you're like me and you just wanna EAT and don't give a shit about appropriate temperature control, toss 'em in hot and add all the fixins. Squirt on the dressing, whip it all around, turn on *Orange is the New Black*, and dig in!

13. Squash-ghetti and Veg-balls — 267 Calories

Prep: 15 minutes
Cook: 45 minutes
Total time: 60 minutes
Yield: Dinner and a doggy bag

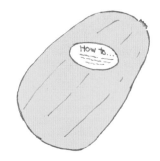

Ingredients
1 cup spaghetti squash "noodles" (42 calories)
5 Morningstar Farms Veggie Meatballs (130 calories)
½ cup Ragu No Sugar Added Tomato Basil Pasta Sauce (60 calories)
1 wedge Laughing Cow Light Creamy Swiss (35 calories)

Directions
For the Squash:
The great (and hilarious) thing about spaghetti squash is that each gargantuan gourd comes with its own "how-to" sticker stuck on. So, for cooking the squash, refer to sticker. The layman's instructions are simple: Cut squash in half length-wise, deseed. Place face-down on a baking sheet and bake for however long the sticker tells you to. I will say that I have nearly dismembered each one of my ten fingers struggling with these monstrous veggie boulders, so have a decent knife (I've never had one) and handle with care. When the glorious nad is fully roasted, let it sit for a good while—that shit's hot. If you are impatient, put on oven mitts for this next part. Take a fork and scrape out the meat in long, downward strokes. See how it's making faux-noodles?!??! So fun! Exciting! Keep scraping till you've gotten every last string out of that sucker. The full squash should yield a good 3–4 servings.

For the Balls:
Microwave Morningstar meatballs. Yay!

For the Creamy Saucy Sauce:
Heat up low calorie marinara in a saucepan. I prefer the Ragu, but have some fun in the marketplace and pick out something different that meets your budget requirements if you like! Once it's hot, plop a wedge or two of Laughing Cow Light Swiss and stir till it melts in for a creamy red sauce effect. (Alkies, must you insist on authentic ala vodka, just take a shot for 60 calories.)

Once everything's ready, throw squash noodles in a bowl, drop meatballs on top, finish with the sauce, and if you need hot sauce (0 calories!) and Parmesan (30 calories per tbsp), do what you will. YUM!

14. Happy Lettuce Wraps — 150 Calories

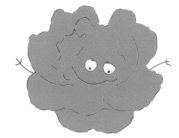

Prep: 10 minutes
Cook: 15 minutes
Total time: 30 minutes
Yield: 4 wraps

Ingredients
"Butter" Pam cooking spray (0 calories)
¼ container firm tofu (88 calories)
4 leaves Bibb lettuce (5 calories)
1 package angel hair shirataki noodles (0 calories)
½ cup shredded red cabbage (14 calories)
½ cup sliced cucumber (8 calories)

½ cup julienned carrots (25 calories)
1 tsp sriracha hot chili sauce (10 calories)

Directions

Omg you guys, these things are so good AND so portable! Take them to work, to a picnic in the park, on the airplane, or to a movie theatre! (For the movies: always remember to crack open secretly smuggled food or drink items during poppy opening credit songs or gun fights/car chases.) Heat up a skillet and spray a BUNCH of Pam (preferably, at least for this concept, butter flavor) all over the sizzle. Add sliced tofu and "fry."* Meanwhile, julienne your veggies and wash and dry your lettuce cups. Cook your smelly shirataki, too.** When everything's ready, line each lettuce cup with noodles, then add sliced tofu. Top with julienned veggies and put as much or as little sriracha on top as you want. (These things come so cheap you might feel like you can roll a little higher. If you can afford it, add a dollop of almond butter to each cup . . . at about 100 calories per tbsp, be sure you can *really* afford it, but you know your budget.) Roll up, arrange in Tupperware, conceal in purse, and enjoy while fawning over the new Zac Efron.

15. Shirataki Miracle Slop — 30 Calories

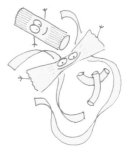

Prep: 1 minute
Cook: 2 minutes

---

* This really just means cook a long time in the Pam and you'll fool yourself into some kind of crusty buttery effect.

** This stuff is going to take the place of vermicelli noodles, but with less (read: ZERO) calories added on. For more about this miracle noodle, see page 71.

Total time: 3 minutes
Yield: 1 bowl of wonder munchies during Jimmy Fallon

Ingredients
1–2 packages shirataki miracle noodles (or 5 packages, who cares!? 0 calories)
I Can't Believe It's Not Butter spray (0 calories)
Louisiana Hot Sauce (0 calories)
1 tbsp grated Parmesan cheese (30 calories)

Okay guys. Three truths:

1. This shit is legitimately a miracle.
2. It's best to eat it late at night, as a drunk/high munchie, so you're not as aware of the hard-to-shake fishy stink.
3. Be mindful if you're able. Sometimes I'm so grossed out by the stank and the thought of the stank, even if the stank ain't there no more, that I just pile on more and more Parmesan cheese to mask the stank, and soon I've added as many calories as if I'd just eaten real noodles. So. Just know what you're getting into.

Directions
Take the package of stink noodles, cut them open, let them pour out into a strainer with all their stank. Rinse with cool water. Meanwhile, put some water on the stove and bring to a boil. When stink noodles are satisfactorily rinsed, boil 'em for 2–3 minutes, until their stink has subsided. (Somewhat. It will never disappear completely.) Once you've extinguished the stink to the best of your ability, strain and dry a bit with a paper towel. Pour I Can't Believe It's Not Butter spray all the hell

over the noodles, and plop squirmy mess in a dish. Smother with hot sauce and Parmesan. Plug your nose and bon appétit!

16. Dix on Stix — 37 Calories per popsicle

Prep: 10 minutes
Inactive: 6 hours-ish
Total time: 6 hours-ish
Yield: 12–16 pops

Ingredients
½ cup lime juice (5 calories)
¼ cup honey (258 calories)
4 cups red grapes, halved (248 calories)
¼ cup fresh mint (5 calories)
2 cups cold water (0 calories)
Popsicle molds!
Popsicle sticks!

Directions
This is something I saw in *Self* magazine once. I'm guessing Julianne Hough was on the cover. These pops are nature's candy, frozen.

Buy popsicle molds. I recommend penis-shaped ones from the Hustler store, because they're hilarious. If you're not feeling funny, I'm sure you can find some less offensive ones at Crate & Barrel or whatever. In a mixing bowl, whisk honey and lime juice till honey dissolves. Stir in water. Stuff penis molds with grapes and mint. Pour liquid over each to fill line. Add sticks (penny pinchers can use twigs from the backyard). Freeze for 6 hours, turn on *Magic Mike*, and suck it.

17. Peachy Green — 114 Calories

Prep: 5 min
Total time: 5 min
Yield: 1 summery salad

Ingredients
1 fresh peach, sliced (38 calories)
1 ripe tomato, sliced (31 calories)
5 leaves basil (0 calories)
2 tbsp Newman's Own Lite Balsamic Vinaigrette (45 calories)

Directions
Take out a peach. Wash it. Slice it. Save the pit for crafting.* Take out a tomato. Wash it. Slice it. Throw peaches and tomatoes in a bowl with basil and top off with Paul Newman. Mix around and chow down! Very guiltless pleasure.

18. Cauliflower-Feta Whip-It — 154 Calories per serving

Prep: 10 minutes
Cook: 30 minutes
Total time: 40 minutes
Yield: impressive cocktail nosh for 4 friendos

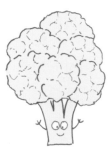

---

* This could be an eventual Christmas tree ornament or the head of a voodoo doll, for example.

Ingredients

8 oz Athenos Fat Free Feta (280 calories)

3 oz Philadelphia Whipped Cream Cheese (193 calories)

1 medium head cauliflower (144 calories)

"Olive Oil" Pam cooking spray (0 calories)

2 tbsp fresh lemon juice (0 calories)

Salt-N-Pepa to taste (0 calories)

It's not like this is terribly low in calories, but it yields a hearty helping, and it's freaking delicious. The roasted cauliflower is a suggestion, and a nice looking hors d'oeuvre at a cocktail party, but you could also just keep the whip-it around for a schmear or a dip with any old thing. You don't necessarily need a food processor for this—you can use a blender or a gaggle of nimble-fingered child laborers—but a food processor is ideal.

Directions

For the Whipped Feta:

Athenos Fat Free Feta comes in crumble or block form. Buy the block to get the most bang for your buck. A great way to measure out your serving size from the block is to cut the whole thing into even sixths—each sixth is an ounce. You're going to want to take 1 whole block and 2 sixths from a second block, crumble it all up, and dump into a food processor. Pulse the crumbles a few times, till they're tiny crumbles. Add 3 oz whipped cream cheese and puree till smooth. There's your whipped feta.

For the Baked Cauliflower:

Preheat oven to 450 degrees. Take a nice looking head of cauliflower. Put it on a cookie sheet. Douse it in olive oil flavored Pam. Squeeze a couple lemons on it. Sprinkle some salt and pepper, and put it in the oven for about 30 minutes. When it comes out, it should be pretty tender—the florets should pull away easily. Serve on a cutesy platter with the whipped feta as a dip, uncork the pinot, bitch about exes, and stuff your faces with creamy cheesy salty goodness.

19. Apple-Bottom Bruschetta — 272 Calories

Prep: 5 minutes
Total time: 5 minutes
Yield: 6–8 lil' apple snacks

Ingredients
1 green apple (80 calories)
¼ cup Sargento Fat Free Ricotta (50 calories)
1 tbsp honey (60 calories)
25 shelled pistachios (82 calories)

Directions
Bruschetta without the bread! Genius!

Slice 1 medium-sized green apple into circles—as many as you can get, each about ½-inch thick. Measure out ¼ cup of the fat free ricotta. Evenly distribute and spread on apple rounds. Do the same with your 1 tablespoon of honey and drizzle evenly atop all the cheese. Put 25 shelled pistachios in a plastic baggie and beat the shit out of them with a hammer or a tennis racket or whatever you have lying around, then sprinkle the crumbs on the apple-ricotta-honey rounds. You've got yourself a delightful treat, and soon you'll no longer be an apple-bottom!

20. Huge Ass Taco Salad — 360 Calories

Prep: 5 minutes
Cook: 10 minutes
Total time: 15 minutes
Yield: 1 really awesome and satisfying dinner

Ingredients
1 package romaine lettuce, chopped (30 calories)
½ cup Smart Ground Mexican Style "taco meat" (120 calories)
¼ cup Kraft Fat Free Shredded Cheddar (45 calories)
¼ cup black beans (55 calories)
2 tbsp Newman's Own Medium Chunky Salsa (10 calories)
3 packets stolen Taco Bell Fire Sauce (0 calories)
1 Doritos 100-calorie pack (100 calories)

You guys. The Chili's "Quesadilla Explosion Salad" (sounds like me in my twenties after a bad breakup) has 1,430 calories. You could have three of these Huge Ass Taco Salads, and the only explosion would be in your pants, from the beans. If you're hungry tonight, I've got just what you need.

Directions
Take the pack of prepared/chopped/washed romaine. Dump it in a big salad bowl. (If you want to buy fresh romaine, wash it, dry it, and chop it yourself, be my guest. But if you are my guest, dining at my house, you will be served bagged romaine. Because I am lazy.) Squeeze fake taco meat onto the skillet and turn up the heat, separating and stirring around till everything's heated. In the meantime, open and drain

your beans. Add 'em to the lettuce. By now the fake meat is heated through—it doesn't need to cook, you'd just prefer it wasn't lukewarm fake meat. Dump it on top of the lettuce and beans. Add cheese, salsa, and Fire Sauce.* To top off with an exciting crunch, crumple a 100-calorie bag of Nacho Cheesier** Doritos to make a bunch of crumbs, then open and pour over your salad. (It's best to go with the 100-calorie bag. If you get a normal or "FAMILY SIZE" bag and just take out 11 chips to crumble, you and I both know the rest of that bag is gonna be gone by the time *Nightline* comes on.)

You've got yourself a taco salad! A huge ass one at that! Olé!

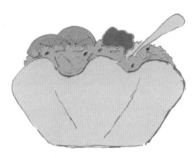

---

* I believe they're now selling this stuff in bottles, but every time I pass a Taco Bell, I run in, throw twenty packs of Fire Sauce and a couple of sporks in my purse, and run away. I'm set for years.

** Cheesier than what?

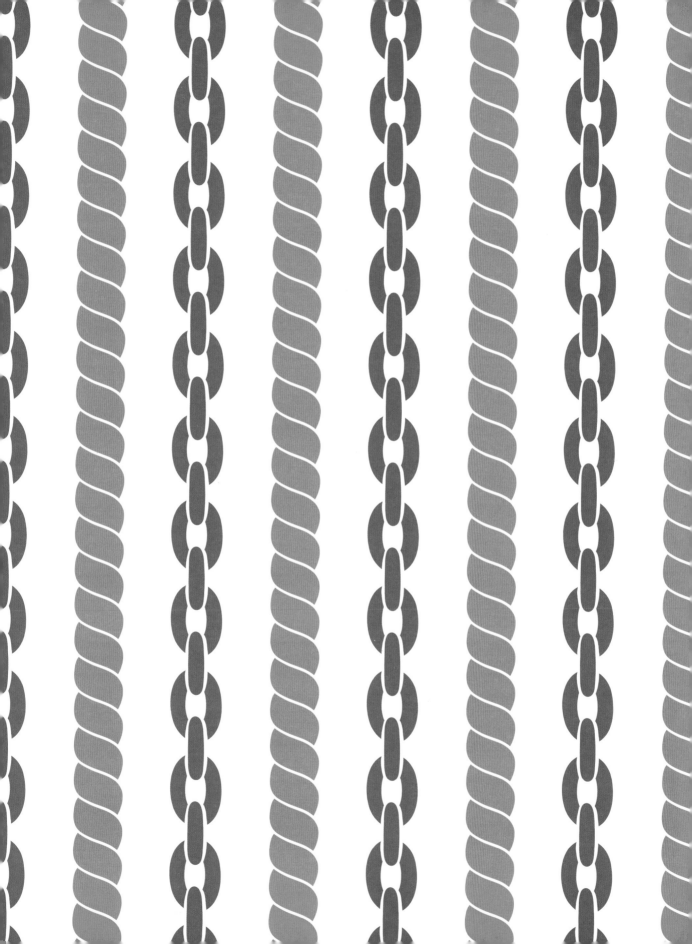

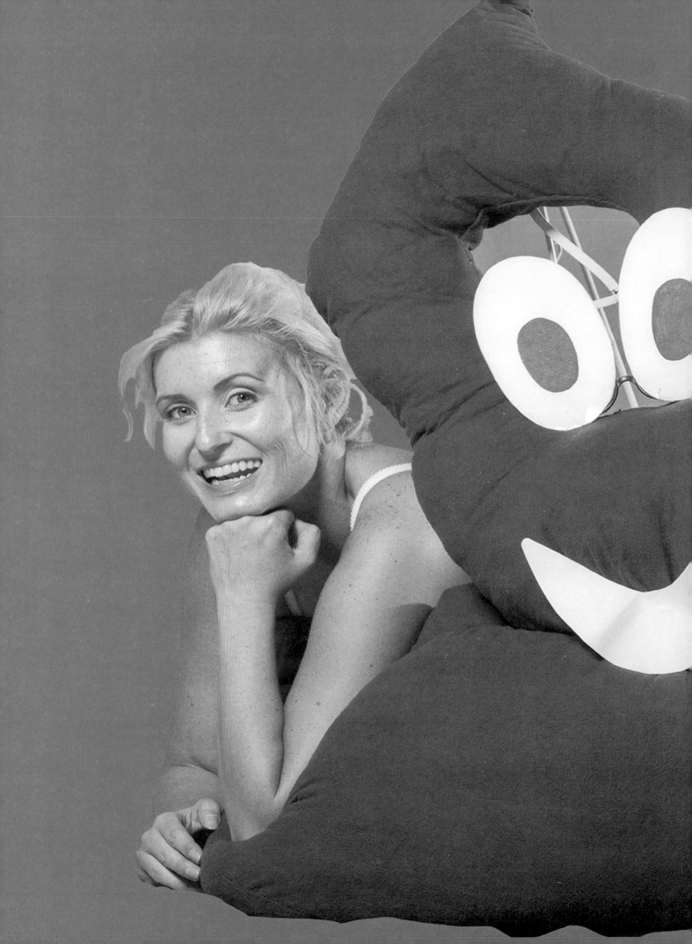

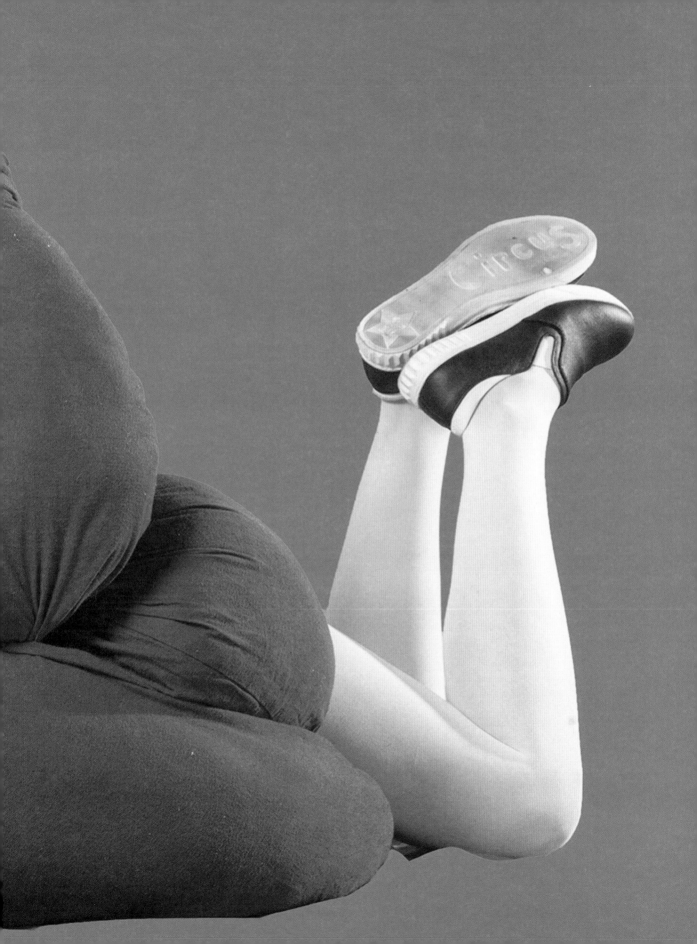

Loser Ledger

	DAY	DATE	WEIGHT	BMR

Time	Food	Cals In	Exercise	Cals Out

| Totals | Add "Cals In" Column → | | Add "Cals Out" Column → | |

Calories In − Calories Out − BMR = Total Net Calories

Loser Ledger

_____ DAY _____ DATE _____ WEIGHT [BMR box] BMR

Time	Food	Cals In	Exercise	Cals Out

| Totals | Add "Cals In" Column → | | Add "Cals Out" Column → | |

Calories In − Calories Out − BMR = Total Net Calories

Loser Ledger

_____ DAY   _____ DATE   _____ WEIGHT   ⬜ BMR

Time	Food	Cals In	Exercise	Cals Out

| Totals | Add "Cals In" Column → | | Add "Cals Out" Column → | |

⬜ Calories In   −   ⬜ Calories Out   −   ⬜ BMR   =   ✺ Total Net Calories

Loser Ledger

DAY _____   DATE _____   WEIGHT _____   BMR [____]

Time	Food	Cals In	Exercise	Cals Out
Totals	Add "Cals In" Column →		Add "Cals Out" Column →	

[Calories In] − [Calories Out] − [BMR] = Total Net Calories

Loser Ledger

DAY _____ DATE _____ WEIGHT _____ BMR [ ]

Time	Food	Cals In	Exercise	Cals Ou

| Totals | Add "Cals In" Column → | | Add "Cals Out" Column → | |

[Calories In] − [Calories Out] − [BMR] = [Total Net Calories]

Loser Ledger

DAY   DATE   WEIGHT   BMR

Time	Food	Cals In	Exercise	Cals Out

| Totals | Add "Cals In" Column → | | Add "Cals Out" Column → | |

Calories In − Calories Out − BMR = Total Net Calories

Index

Acknowledgments

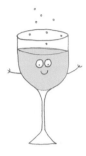

That was awesome.

The book, I mean.

Right? Wasn't it? I think so.

You know why it was awesome?

Because these people are awesome:

Mom and Dad, thanks for being the best, which is also, so very often, the worst. You have always been so spectacularly annoying and obnoxious, so all-up-in-my-shit and opinionated, so readily averse to everything that excites me, so consistently in accordance with everything I hate. You are the omniscient and ubiquitous moral and directional compasses of my life, no matter how old I become, no matter how far away I live from home, no matter what I do, no matter how I might try to escape and call myself an independent woman once and for all—you are the nagging voices in my head that won't ever go away. Nor will your porch calls. And

I'm grateful for that. You've kept me young; I'm forever an angsty teen. Because as much as I snap and whine and complain and know it all, without your constant harassment, I'd be a shell of myself. I love you both so so so so much. Thank you for the fun and the funny.

And a million thanks to Betsy Levy, too (Mom's professional alter ego), for being the best darn illustrator a girl could ask for, and at an unbeatable price! Your meticulous and schlubby drawings were all perfect in my book (literally), and I really think you could/should consider a part-time job as a caricaturist, or at least just a Billy Joel portraitist.

Sam and Erica Levy, your sisterly support and uncensored feedback is always a blessing, even when delivered amid many a curse. Let's sister-trip again soon. Extra thanks in advance to my agent Samantha Levy (another familial and delusional alter ego), who will, by now, have scheduled out a fantastic American Summer Book Tour that I am SO excited about!! (If this has not yet materialized and I have to figure out the whole goddamn thing by myself, you can kiss your 10% goodbye. But regardless, in humbled appreciation for your phenomenal proofreading skills and your jackpot vision for the pitted-out gym pics, that Winnebago's going nowhere without you.)

Billy Hot Chocolate. Slim. Stretch. Mister Softee. Mister Boyfriend. Mister Parker. Mister Mandy-Levy-Social-Media and Mister Proofreader-Number-Two. Mister Ben Wyatt, as far as I'm concerned. I don't mean to be a total queeah, but I love you, and you have made me the best version of myself, and we're a real team, and you get me, and you call me on my bullshit, and you hold me accountable, and you teach me about Catholics, and you shower me with snacks, and you hate my run-on sentences, and I think you are so smart and so funny and so kind, and every stranger that you meet is happy to know you, and getting to be loved by you makes me the luckiest gal in the world, and I can't wait to hang out with you forever! Okay now I'm going to do an armpit fart because I'm making myself gag!

A billion thanks to Caroline Knecht, the scrappiest book editor in all of New York City: Did you ever know that you're my hero? Praise Jesus for 'knechting' us over jello shots and *Strangers with Candy*. If not for your enthusiasm, know-how, mutual obsession with (predominantly guilt-ily pleasurable) pop culture, expertly executed email correspondence, unworldly anime eyes, witty one-liners and crude asides, and a natural knack for pacifying and reassuring an anxiety-ridden control freak, none of this would have been possible, and I'd be eating double the cheese that I do today. You are a pro and a friend. I'm so happy this project brought us together.

To Melinda and Lacey, The Sisters Voss, I am sincerely sorry for the ways in which I use and abuse your endless talents and unstoppably creative minds, but I just can't help it; after all, you are willing workhorses from an Ohio farm and I am eternally grateful for the sunshine and amaz-ingness that you girls and your wonderful family have brought into my life. Thank you for being there through thick and thin (read: the various physical iterations of Mandy), for being hilarious, for being excited, for being the most able bitches I know. Between the two of you, you styled and designed my photo shoot, were grips and PAs to our photog, han-dled hair and makeup, made a dress out of lettuce, and pumped my veins with Diet Coke at every whispering inkling of a diva breakdown. And all the while you smiled. And fucking crushed it. I love you girls.

And a lifetime of indebtedness to the enormously talented Christopher Patrick Ernst, Frumpie-Frump, CPE, our master photographer and aesthetic visionary. You are a godsend, an artist, and a delight, and hot DAMN do you have a nice vintage furniture/furnishings collection! (Special shout-out to Lilli Albin for knowing he'd be perfect for the gig and connecting us—high five out to Austin, Lilli!) But really Christopher, thank you so much for your brilliant eye, spot-on ideas, insane generosity and hospitality, and perplexingly chill disposition throughout the course of a seventy-two-hour shoot teeming with estrogen and the shrillest of sister-fights. Your photos are gorgeous and more perfect than anything I ever could have imagined. I love my book because of your work. Thank you. :)

To Shell & Shag at 94 Jewel Street—your studio rocks and so do you! Thanks for having us! To everyone at Skyhorse, thank you so much for taking a chance on me—I swear to God I will not disappoint! I hope I can be your next Jenna Jameson. To Chipotle for helping me get fat; to Chop't for helping me get thin. To Cincinnati and to LA. I love and miss you both. To Projectmill: keep doing cool shit. To Jenny Lewis for being my steady idol. To Ferris Bueller for being my first love. To Lesley, to Becky, to Beth, to Adam, to Cindy, to Josh, to Ken, to Sean the Cat and Ginny, too. To the Beatles. And not to the Stones.

LY, darling dears. On to the next one!

-M

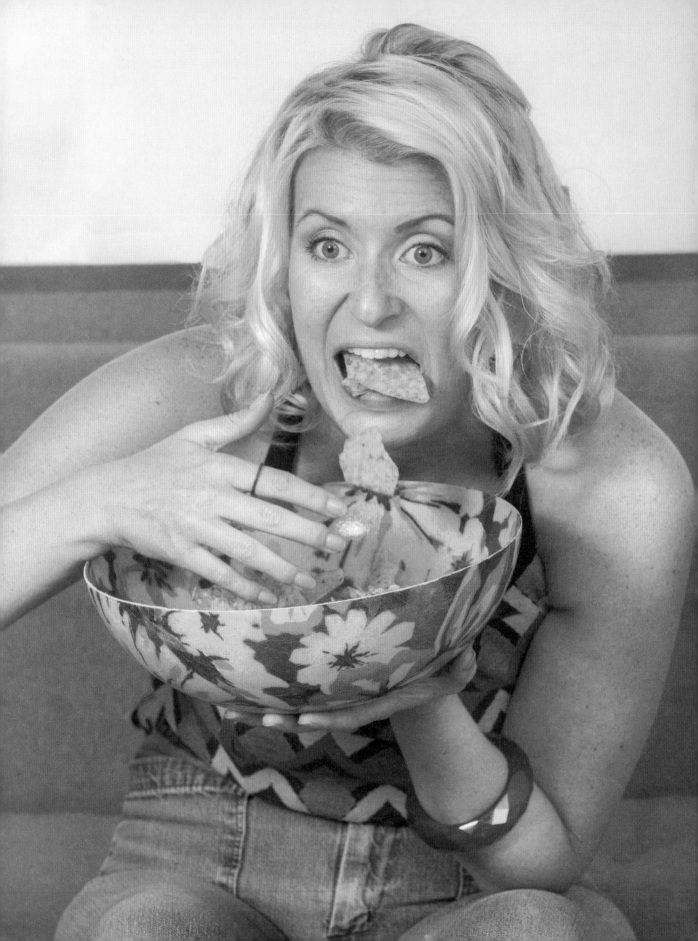

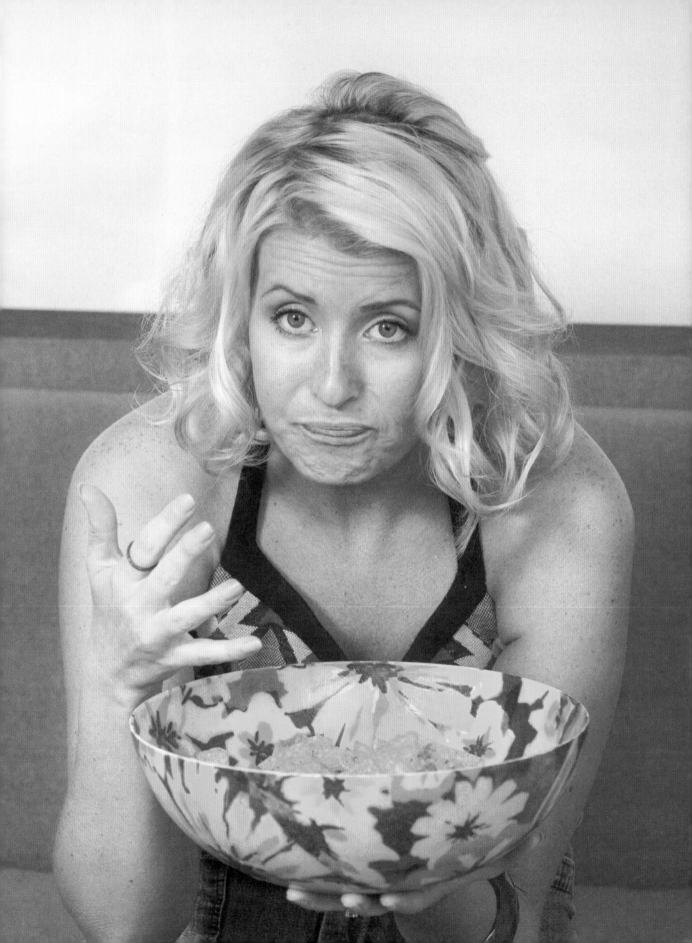

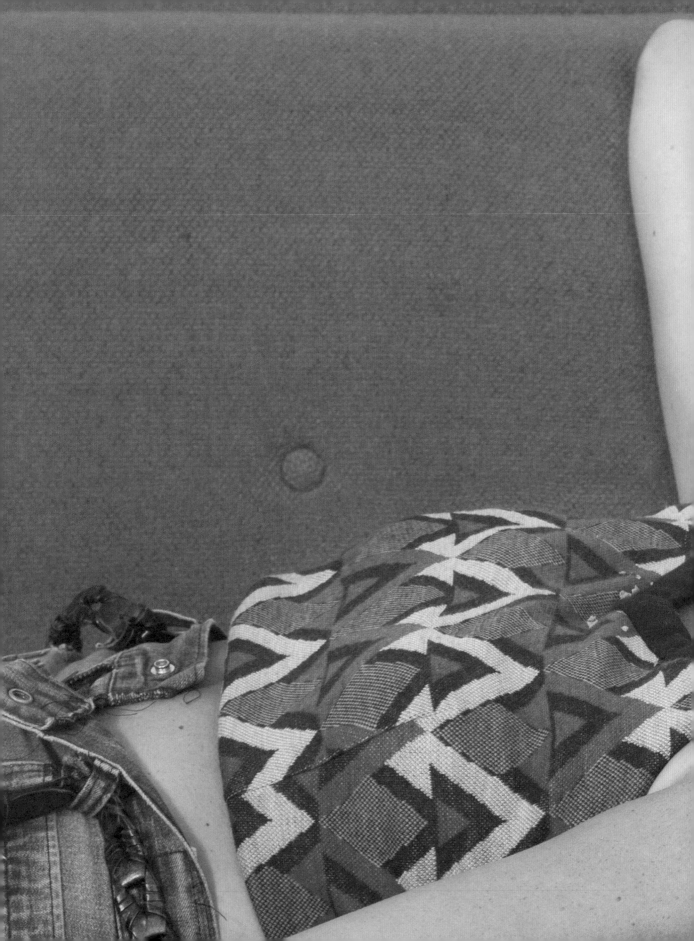

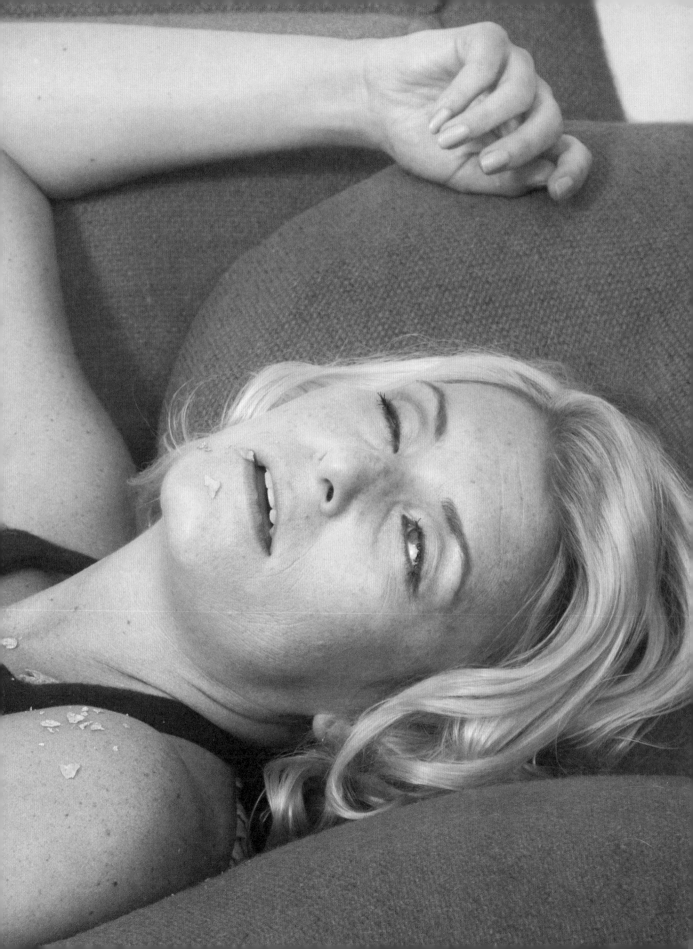

Masks!

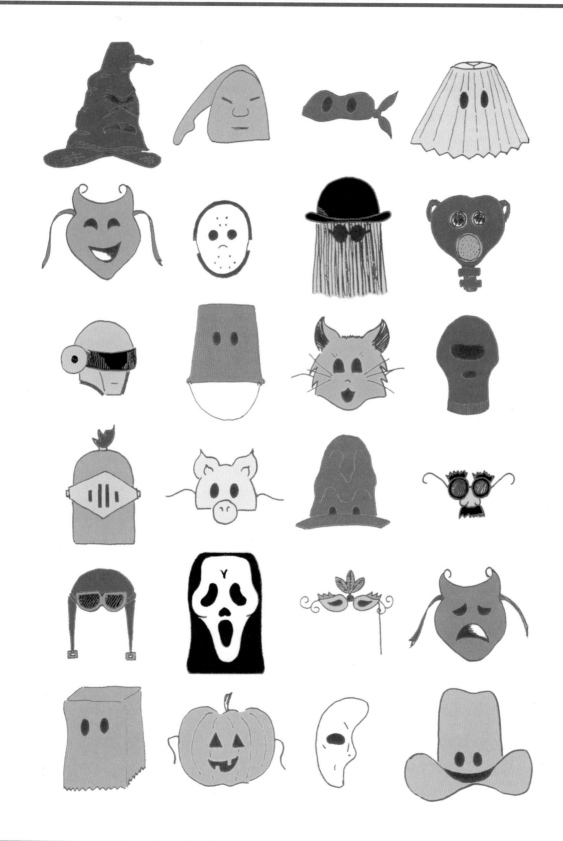

Masks!

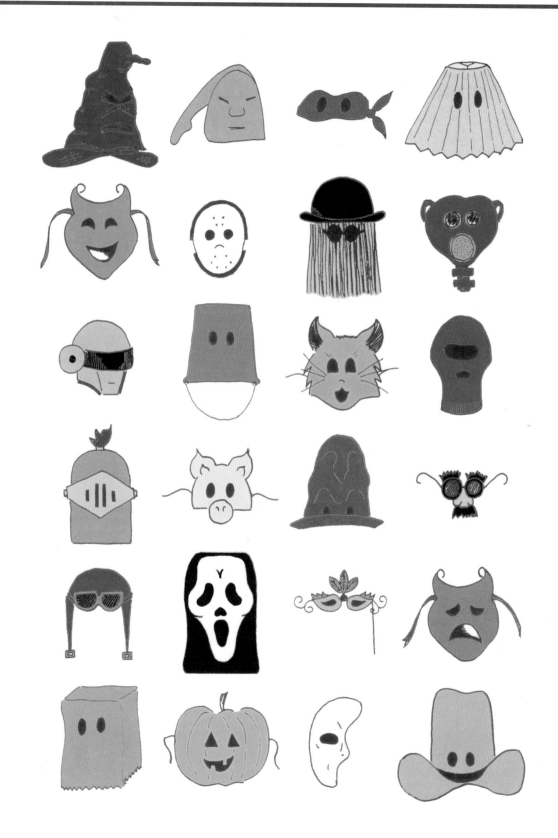

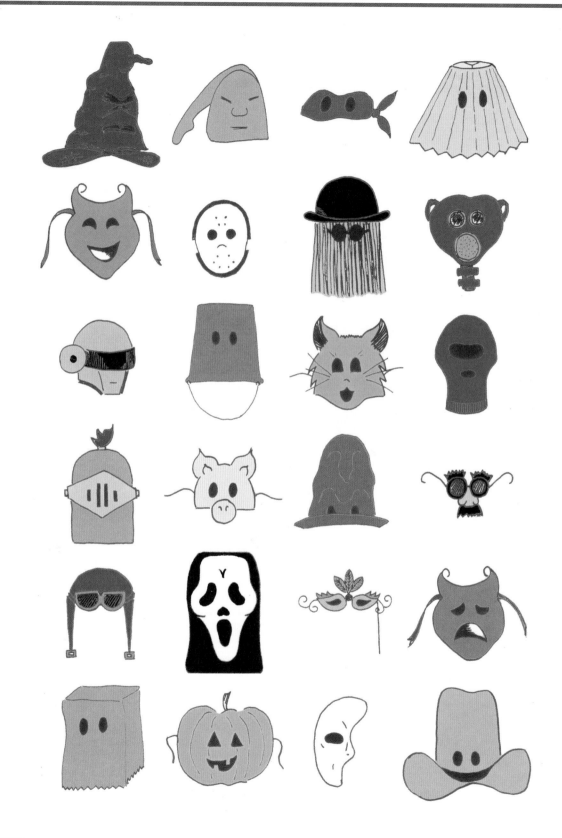